How to Implement Evidence-Based Healthcare

T0254095

Dedication

In memory of Anna Donald. I have finally finished our book.

How to Implement Evidence-Based Healthcare

Trisha Greenhalgh
Professor of Primary Care Health Sciences
Nuffield Department of Primary Care Health Sciences
University of Oxford
Oxford, UK

WILEY Blackwell

This edition first published 2018
© 2018 John Wiley & Sons Ltd.

Registered Offices
John Wiley & Sons, Inc., 111 River Street, Hoboken, NJ 07030, USA
John Wiley & Sons Ltd., The Atrium, Southern Gate, Chichester, West Sussex, PO19 8SQ, UK

Editorial Office
9600 Garsington Road, Oxford, OX4 2DQ, UK

For details of our global editorial offices, customer services, and more information about Wiley products visit us at www.wiley.com.

Wiley also publishes its books in a variety of electronic formats and by print-on-demand. Some content that appears in standard print versions of this book may not be available in other formats.

Library of Congress Cataloging-in-Publication data are available

ISBN: 9781119238522

Cover image: Meaden Creative
Cover design by Wiley

Set in 9.5/12pt Minion by SPi Global, Pondicherry, India

Printed in the UK

Contents

Foreword

Starting to read the new book by Trisha Greenhalgh on the implementation of evidence-based healthcare (EBHC), I remembered one of the major implementation projects in healthcare in the Netherlands, in which I was involved in the 1990s. A national collaboration between the Department of Health and the GP organisations aimed at improving prevention in primary care by implementing national guidelines for flu vaccination, cervical screening and cardiovascular risk reduction. My team developed the implementation programmme and studied the impact. We developed a programme at different levels of healthcare (national, local, practice, professional) using a variety of theories on implementing change, including the setting of evidence-based guidelines, education for professionals, educational materials for patients, a national steering group, outreach visitors to support practices, a fee for the extra work, etc. The results were great: an enormous increase in vaccination and screening rates in a very short time. However, within 3 years the project stopped, because of a political fight between the GP organisations and the Department of Health over both the aims of the programme (more or less primary prevention) and general policies and honoraria for primary care. It took years before prevention was put on the agenda of primary care again.

There were many lessons in this project that I will never forget, even though it is 20 years ago and I retired from scientific work a while ago. For instance, the impact of political support on effective change, but also the role of professional attitude to the change required (many GPs were quite reluctant to primary prevention). Reading this new book by one of our absolute experts in the field of implementation of change in healthcare, I understand the successes and failures of this project even better. EBHC and evidence-based guidelines do not implement themselves, even if the evidence is sound. Many policy-makers and professionals sometimes have naive ideas about the implementation of change in practice. Ineffective implementation of EBHC is, most of the time, a waste of time and money. Implementation of change in healthcare is, most of the time, only successful when you work at different levels of healthcare, not only at the level of professionals, and when you use sound theories and assumptions to guide your efforts.

Exactly these messages you will find in this very interesting and useful book. It is rich in ideas and provides a whole range of theories. It makes clear how important it is to use knowledge and theories from different sources, including social and political sciences and humanities. The author wrote the book in the memory of her friend, Anna Donald. Together they started with the idea of the book back in the 1990s, but only now has the author been able to work on it and finish it. A great achievement, which demonstrates how this complex field of implementation of EBHC has developed over the years and has come to maturity over the past decades. Please read the book and use it in your programmes and projects.

Professor Richard Grol,
Emeritus Professor on Quality of Care;
Founder and former Director of the Scientific Institute on Quality of Healthcare

Acknowledgements

To the late Dr Anna Donald, for beginning this journey with me (see Chapter 1 for the full story).

To my students, for asking the awkward questions that inspired much of this book.

To the many colleagues in – and especially beyond – the world of academia, for introducing me to different perspectives.

To everyone on Twitter who contributed suggestions.

To my family (Fraser, Rob, Al) for being cool about this writing habit of mine – and chipping in occasionally.

To the doctors and nurses who saved my life last year (using NICE guidelines).

To everyone at Wiley who supported the development, preparation, publication and sale of this book.

To Gaby Leuenberger for proofreading the manuscript.

Chapter 1 **Introduction**

1.1 The story of this book

Let me start with a warning: this book is not going to give you a cookbook answer to the question of how to implement evidence-based healthcare (EBHC). My (more modest) aim is threefold:

1. To introduce you to different ways of thinking about the evidence, people, organisations, technologies and so on (read the chapter headings) that are relevant to the challenge of implementing EBHC.
2. To persuade you that implementing EBHC is not an exact science and can never be undertaken in a formulaic, algorithmic way. Rather – and notwithstanding all the things that are known to help or hinder the process – it will always require contextual judgement, rules of thumb, instinct and perhaps a lucky alignment of circumstances.
3. To promote interest in the social sciences (e.g. sociology, social psychology, anthropology) and humanities (e.g. philosophy, literature/storytelling, design) as the intellectual basis for many of the approaches described in this book.

This book was a long time in gestation. The idea first came to Anna Donald and me in the late 1990s. At the time, we were both working in roles that involved helping people and organisations implement evidence – and it was proving a lot harder than the textbooks of the time implied. That was the decade in which evidence-based medicine (EBM), which later expanded beyond the exclusive realm of doctors to EBHC (to include the activities of other health professionals, managers and lay people), was depicted as a straightforward sequence of asking a clinical question, searching the literature for relevant research articles, critically appraising those articles and implementing the findings. The last task in the sequence was depicted as something that could be ticked off from a checklist.

How to Implement Evidence-Based Healthcare, First Edition. Trisha Greenhalgh.
© 2018 John Wiley & Sons Ltd. Published 2018 by John Wiley & Sons Ltd.

Anna and I penned an outline for the book (it looked very different then – because most of the research into knowledge translation and implementation cited here had not yet been done). But, tragically, Anna became ill before we got much further and died a few years later, with our magnum opus barely started. Whilst the detail of what is described here is my own work, there is still a sense in which it is Anna's work too. Even in those early days, before terms like 'implementation science', 'research utilisation', 'knowledge translation' and 'evidence-into-action' became part of our vocabulary, Anna recognised that we would never be able to produce a set of evidence implementation checklists in the same way as she and I once drew up a set of critical appraisal checklists for our students.

It has taken me nearly 20 years to produce this book, partly because when Anna died, I lost a dear friend as well as a formidable intellectual sparring partner – but also because the question 'How do you implement EBHC?' is a good deal too broad for a single book. And yet, *one* book to scope the field and run a narrative through its many dimensions was exactly what was needed. I have long been convinced that whilst there are definite advantages to asking dozens of different authors, each with different views on the subject, to cover different aspects of this complex and contested field (Sharon Straus and her team did just that, and the book they edited is worth reading [1]), the EBHC community (nay, network of communities) also needs a single-author textbook whose goal is to achieve some degree of coherence across the disparate topics.

EBM and EBHC have come a long way since the 1990s. The 'campaign for real EBM', which I helped establish in 2014, has called for a broadening of EBM's parameters to include the use of social science methodologies to study the nuances of clinical practice, policymaking and the patient experience – as well as considering the political dimension of conflicts of interest in research funding and industry sponsorship of trials [2]. It is, perhaps, a reflection of the broadening of the EBM/EBHC agenda that implementation science has been established as a separate interdisciplinary field of inquiry (with much internal contestation), with its own suite of journals, research funding panels and conference circuit [3].

One important development in EBHC in recent years is the growing emphasis on value for money in the research process and an emerging evidence base on how little impact research so often has on practice and policy. This overlaps with the expectation on universities (in the United Kingdom at least, via the Research Excellence Framework) to demonstrate that the research they undertake has impact beyond publishing papers in journals read only by other academics. I have reviewed the literature on research impact elsewhere [4].

In 2014, Sir Iain Chalmers led a series in the *Lancet* that highlighted different aspects of research waste, including waste in the allocation of research funds (too often, we study questions people don't want answered and fail to study the ones they do) [5]; waste in the conduct of research (studies are underpowered, use the wrong primary endpoints and/or the wrong measurements and so on) [6]; and waste when the findings of research prove 'unusable' in practice (because the findings are not presented in ways that could be applied by practitioners or policymakers) [7]. Most recently, John Ioannidis has written a masterly review on 'Why Most Clinical Research Is Not Useful' [8]. I look at this last paper in detail in Section 9.1. The bottom line is clear: there is a huge gap between evidence and its implementation – and it's not easily explained.

The final impetus for me finishing this book was taking up a new job at the University of Oxford in 2015. My new job description included leading (along with Kamal Mahtani) the module 'Knowledge Into Action'. This was part of the popular and well-regarded MSc in Evidence-Based Health Care run by Carl Heneghan and his team from the Centre for Evidence-Based Medicine. The students on the Knowledge Into Action course were asking for a textbook. Some (the less experienced ones) were looking for checklists and formulae – but many who had worked at the interface between evidence and practice for years knew that the field was not predictable enough to be solved by such things. These more enlightened students wanted a way to get their heads round *why* implementing EBHC is not an exact science.

In sum, this book looks two ways. Looking retrospectively, it is dedicated to the memory of Anna Donald, who helped inspire it. And looking prospectively, it is dedicated to those who study the implementation of EBHC with a view to improving outcomes for patients. It also seeks to make a contribution to increasing value and reducing waste in research by increasing the proportion of good research that has a worthwhile impact on patients (the sick) and on citizens (including those of us who pay taxes and who may become sick).

1.2 There is no tooth fairy ...

This section started life as a blog on the website of the Centre for Evidence Based Health Care at the University of Oxford. I wrote it to set the scene for the Knowledge Into Action MSc module that Kamal Mahtani and I were running in 2016. Our group of students had already completed modules on critical appraisal, randomised controlled trials and other highly rigorous methodological approaches. They perhaps anticipated that 'rigorous methodology' would get them through the implementation stage too. To get my excuses in before the course began, I penned this blog entry:

> Tools and resources for critical appraisal of research evidence are widely available and extremely useful. Whatever the topic and whatever the study design used to research it, there is probably a checklist to guide you step by step through assessing its validity and relevance.
>
> The implementation challenge is different. Let me break this news to you gently: there is no tooth fairy. Nor is there any formal framework or model or checklist of things to do (or questions to ask) that will take you systematically through everything you need to do to 'implement' a particular piece of evidence in a particular setting.
>
> There are certainly tools available [see Appendices], and you should try to become familiar with them. They will prompt you to adapt your evidence to suit a local context, identify local 'barriers' and 'facilitators' to knowledge use, select and tailor your interventions, and monitor and evaluate your progress. All these aspects of implementation are indeed important.
>
> But here's the rub: despite their value, knowledge-to-action tools cannot be applied mechanistically in the same way as the CONSORT checklist [2] can be applied to a paper describing a randomised controlled trial. This is not because the tools are in some way flawed (in which case, the solution would be to refine the tools, just as people have refined the CONSORT checklist over the years). It is because implementation is infinitely more complex (and hence unpredictable) than a research study in which confounding variables have been (or should have been) controlled or corrected for.
>
> Implementing research evidence is not just a matter of following procedural steps. You will probably relate to that statement if you've ever tried it, just as you may know as a parent that raising a child is not just a matter of reading and applying the child-rearing manual, or as a tennis player that winning a match cannot be achieved merely by knowing the rules of tennis and studying detailed statistics on your opponent's performance in previous games. All these are examples of **complex practices** that require skill and situational judgement (which comes from experience) as well as evidence on 'what works'.
>
> So-called 'implementation science' is, in reality, not a science at all – nor is it an art. It is a **science-informed practice**. And just as with child-rearing and tennis-playing, you get better at it by doing two things in addition to learning about 'what works': doing it, and sharing stories about doing it with others who are also doing it. By reflecting carefully on your own practice and by discussing real case examples shared by others,

*you will acquire not just the abstract knowledge about 'what works' but also the practical wisdom that will help you make contextual judgements about **what is likely to work** (or at least, what might be tried out to see if it works) in **this situation** for **these people** in **this organisation** with **these constraints**.*

There is a philosophical point here. Much healthcare research is oriented to producing statistical generalisations based on one population sample to predict what will happen in a comparable sample. In such cases, there is usually a single correct interpretation of the findings. In contrast, implementation science is at least partly about using unique case examples as a window to wider truths through the enrichment of understanding (what philosophers of science call 'naturalistic generalisation'). In such cases, multiple interpretations of a case are possible and there may be no such thing as the 'correct' answer (recall the example of raising a child above).

In the Knowledge Into Action module, some of the time will be spent on learning about conceptual tools such as the Knowledge to Action Framework [see Appendix A]. But the module is deliberately designed to expose students to detailed case examples that offer multiple different interpretations. We anticipate that at least as much learning will occur as students not only apply 'tools' but also bring their rich and varied life experience (as healthcare professionals, policymakers, managers and service users) to bear on the case studies presented by their fellow students and visiting speakers. Students will also have an opportunity to explore different interpretations of their chosen case in a written assignment.

I hope this blog entry has conveyed the inherent complexity and uncertainty of the field I will be exploring in this book. If you are interested in attending the Knowledge Into Action course, google 'Oxford MSc in Evidence Based Health Care' and find it on the list of modules. The residential week usually runs in late spring, when Oxford is at its glorious best – but be warned: the course usually books up several months in advance.

1.3 Outline of this book

As you can see from the list of chapter titles, each chapter looks at a different level of analysis. Separating the world out into different levels is a useful analytic technique but is in danger of introducing an artificial sense of order. Any attempt to implement EBHC in real life will require you to consider the material from more than one chapter (and ideally all the chapters) in combination.

Chapter 2 looks at evidence. It begins by problematising the very word 'evidence' and encourages you to question the provenance, completeness, relevance and ways of interpreting a piece of evidence – even when it is a randomised controlled trial or systematic review that appears to tick all the right methodological boxes. It also explains the term 'knowledge translation' and reminds you that different users of evidence (researchers, policymakers, practitioners, managers, patients, citizens) come from different cultural 'worlds' and have different values and expectations. It also considers the attributes of evidence (a guideline, for example) that tend to promote its adoption in practice. I offer some tips for generating the kind of evidence that potential users are likely to find useful.

Chapter 3 is about people – all people, since it covers the discipline of psychology, but mainly clinicians, since it relates to the adoption and non-adoption of evidence-based guidelines. I offer a highly eclectic selection of theories of human behaviour, notably 'fast' and 'slow' thinking and the science of heuristics (Kahneman, Gigerenzer); the theory of planned behaviour (Ajzen and Fishbein) and critiques thereof; learning domains of knowledge, skills and attitudes (Bloom); adult learning theory (Kolb, Knowles); social learning theory and self-efficacy (Bandura); and dynamic or staged theories (e.g. Prochaska and DiClemente's stages of change, Rogers' stages of adoption). I also summarise some reviews and empirical studies of why clinicians do not always follow evidence-based guidelines, including work by Michael Cabana, Susan Michie and Richard Grol. I consider empirical evidence from interventions intended to change clinician behaviour – including interventions that prompt, reward or feed back on behaviour; interventions that seek to improve knowledge; interventions that promote the use of heuristics; interventions that promote adult (on-the-job) learning; interventions that promote social influence; and interventions aimed at influencing the stages of change. In a final section, I offer some tips for those who seek to change clinicians' behaviour.

Chapter 4 is about groups and teams. It emphasises the team-based nature of much clinical care these days, and presents evidence on what makes a group or team effective (and, by implication, what may make one ineffective). I contrast different models of leadership – including hierarchical, democratic and distributed; and I suggest, provocatively perhaps, that there are 'male' and 'female' leadership styles (although the former can be adopted by women and the latter by men). I emphasise the importance of facilitation, and introduce organisational learning theory (Argyris and Schön). I give some examples of empirical studies of leadership and facilitation. By way of a summary, I offer tips for leading and facilitating your team to implement best evidence.

Chapter 5 considers organisations. Most of the chapter summarises a systematic review my team published in 2004–05 on the diffusion of innovations in healthcare organisations, which has been widely cited and used.

I introduce various components of our diffusion of innovations model in turn, including structural features of the organisation, its propensity to take up new knowledge (*absorptive capacity*) and the presence or not of a *receptive context for change* (including things like organisational culture and climate); the organisation's readiness to adopt a particular innovation (including innovation-system fit); the process of assimilation (i.e. the organisation's initial efforts to take up the innovation); how the innovation is implemented within the organisation; the external ('outer') context, including the behaviour of other organisations in the same sector; and the dynamic linkage between all these elements. The chapter also includes the findings from a later update to our original diffusion of innovations review, covering the routinisation and sustainability of complex service-level innovations. I suggest some tips for promoting organisational innovativeness.

Chapter 6 looks at citizens – that is, lay people who are not currently patients. This chapter is about the involvement of citizens in the research process: why it is a good idea to involve them (and why it will help the implementation of best practice); how to avoid tokenism; how to 'co-create' research with citizens and communities; and how to communicate the findings of research to a lay audience. I summarise with some tips on how to improve patient and public involvement in your own research.

Chapter 7 is about patients – that is, all of us when we are sick or in need of care, or believe ourselves to be so. I take a hard look at whether the EBHC community is (or ever has been) 'biased' against patients – in the sense that it has (with the best of intentions) served a researcher or clinician agenda at the expense of the needs of the sick patient. I look at the evidence on implementing evidence with patients in the clinical encounter ('shared decision-making'), drawing heavily on the work of Glyn Elwyn. I also look at the literature on self-management of chronic illness and consider two framings of such management ('biomedical' and 'lifeworld'). I look at patient involvement in service improvement efforts. I then offer some tips for improving evidence-based patient care.

Chapter 8 addresses technology. It begins by trying to bust the myth of technological determinism (i.e. by explaining why technologies do not, in and of themselves, *cause* change). It looks at the expanding industry of medical apps (downloadable pieces of software intended to help the clinician and/or the patient implement evidence in clinical care). Acknowledging that a high proportion of technology projects in healthcare fail, I spend a lot of time discussing the non-adoption and abandonment of technologies by both patients and clinicians. I finish with some tips for using technologies to implement evidence.

Chapter 9 is about policy. I take issue with the research tradition of identifying barriers and facilitators to the use of research evidence in policy, arguing that we first need to understand what policymaking *is*. I describe some theories of how policymaking actually happens (I like to define it as the struggle over ideas). I introduce Carol Weiss's taxonomy of how evidence is used in this struggle – including the instrumental and tactical use of evidence in the rhetorical game of influencing significant stakeholders. Much of this game is about the use of language and 'social drama'. I introduce the terms 'value based healthcare' (Sir Muir Gray) and 'values based healthcare, (Mike Kelly and colleagues), and propose that facts and values are not (as is sometimes assumed in the EBHC world) separate and separable. Rather, the 'facts' of EBHC are irredeemably value-laden. I end with some tips for getting closer alignment between research and policy.

In Chapter 10, I talk about networks. Networks are important because knowledge is more social and more fluid than we often assume. Knowledge (both explicit and tacit) is generated, negotiated, refined and circulated in networks of various kinds. Specifically, I consider social networks and social influence (beginning with Coleman et al.'s classic 1964 study of how Pfizer discovered the power of social influence in drug prescribing); professional communities of practice (and the concept of clinical 'mindlines' developed by John Gabbay and Andrée Le May); and patient communities (especially online support groups for chronic illness). I give some tips for improving networks and networking.

Chapter 11 is about systems. It introduces the concept of complex adaptive systems (which Paul Plsek and I wrote about in a *BMJ* series some years ago). Complex systems are unpredictable and emergent, so they do not lend themselves well to rational planning and rigid milestones. Rather, they need an emergent approach in which there is careful collection of, and response to, emerging data. In this chapter, I also cover realist evaluation and review actor-networks and multi-stakeholder health research systems. My final tips are for working effectively with complex systems.

With practical applications in mind, Appendix A provides an overview of frameworks, tools and techniques, including driver diagrams, process mapping, stakeholder mapping, plan–do–study–act cycles and many more. Appendix B details many (although not all) of the different psychological theories of behaviour change.

One final introductory point: this book is not a comprehensive overview of every aspect of implementing EBHC (any more than a manual on child-rearing could possibly cover every challenge a parent might face). Different authors would have put different things in – and left different things out – from the topics I selected. The ones I cover in this book are the ones I personally think are important and the ones I feel confident to cover. I write it as an introduction to a complex, interdisciplinary and rapidly expanding field of inquiry on which there is (thankfully) no firm consensus. If you want to go beyond one person's perspective on this field, I recommend that you explore beyond the topics covered in this book. A good place to start might be the journal *Implementation Science* (www.implementationscience. biomedcentral.com), which is freely available online, or two key books *Knowledge Translation in Health Care*, edited by Sharon Straus and colleagues [1] and *Improving Patient Care: The implementation of Change in Healthcare* [9].

References

1. Straus, S., Tetroe, J., & Graham, I.D. (2013). *Knowledge Translation in Health Care: Moving from Evidence to Practice*. Chichester, John Wiley & Sons.
2. Schulz, K.F., Altman, D.G., & Moher, D. (2010). CONSORT 2010 statement: updated guidelines for reporting parallel group randomized trials. *Annals of Internal Medicine*, **152**(11), 726–732.
3. Bauer, M.S., Damschroder, L., Hagedorn, H., Smith, J., & Kilbourne, A.M. (2015). An introduction to implementation science for the non-specialist. *BMC Psychology*, **3**, 32.
4. Greenhalgh, T., Raftery, J., Hanney, S., & Glover, M. Research impact: a narrative review. *BMC Medicine*, **14**(1), 78.
5. Chalmers, I., Bracken, M.B., Djulbegovic, B., Garattini, S., Grant, J., Gülmezoglu, A.M., et al. (2014). How to increase value and reduce waste when research priorities are set. *Lancet*, **383**(9912), 156–165.
6. Ioannidis, J.P., Greenland, S., Hlatky, M.A., Khoury, M.J., Macleod, M.R., Moher, D., et al. (2014). Increasing value and reducing waste in research design, conduct, and analysis. *Lancet (London, England)*, **383**(9912), 166–175.
7. Glasziou, P., Altman, D.G., Bossuyt, P., Boutron, I., Clarke, M., Julious, S., et al. (2014). Reducing waste from incomplete or unusable reports of biomedical research. *Lancet*, **383**(9913), 267–276.
8. Ioannidis, J.P. (2016). Why most clinical research is not useful. *PLOS Medicine*, **13**(6), e1002049.
9. Grol, R., Wensing, M., Eccles, M., & Davis, D. (Eds.). (2013). *Improving patient care: the implementation of change in health care*. Oxford, John Wiley & Sons.

Chapter 2 **Evidence**

2.1 (Research) Evidence

This chapter is about evidence (by which, for the purposes of this book, I mean *research* evidence) and its translation. I want to start by problematising the very notion of evidence.

Research findings – published in academic journals, synthesised in systematic reviews and distilled into guidelines – even when they appear to be of the highest quality, are almost always incomplete, ambiguous and contested. And they usually address a problem that is one step removed from the one that needs solving. This is partly because research studies contain numerous methodological flaws [1] – but also because, even when studies are not seriously flawed, science is inherently uncertain.

Take, for example, SPRINT (the Systolic Blood Pressure Intervention Trial), which compared tight versus not-so-tight blood pressure control in people at high risk of cardiovascular events but without diabetes. Its preliminary results were published in the *New England Journal of Medicine* in November 2015 [2]. The trial recruited 9361 people with a mean age of 68 years. The research question (paraphrased) was, 'Should we aim for a systolic blood pressure target of 120 (intervention arm) rather than 140 (control arm) mmHg in people at high risk of heart attack or stroke?' Over a median period of 39 months, participants in the intervention arm experienced a significant reduction in death and cardiovascular events compared to those in the control arm – so much so that the trial was stopped early by the data-monitoring committee.

The SPRINT trial ticked most if not all of the boxes for a methodologically robust clinical trial. It was adequately powered (i.e. big enough) to ensure that if there were a clinically significant effect, differences in outcomes between the groups would be statistically significant. Randomisation was double blind, with identical placebos. Appropriate statistical tests (I was told) were used. And so on. Extrapolating from the findings, commentators

How to Implement Evidence-Based Healthcare, First Edition. Trisha Greenhalgh.
© 2018 John Wiley & Sons Ltd. Published 2018 by John Wiley & Sons Ltd.

concluded that tight control of high blood pressure in people of comparable cardiovascular risk to those in the SPRINT trial could save thousands of lives per year in the United States alone. Coverage in the medical and lay press for the study included such terms as 'landmark', 'groundbreaking', 'obviously worthwhile' (i.e. it was obviously worthwhile to treat blood pressure aggressively in this group) and '120 is the new 140'.

Yet, despite strong evidence for significant potential impact on mortality, criticisms of SPRINT emerged within hours of its publication. The authors, said critics, had focused entirely on the alleged benefits of tight blood pressure control without taking full account of the potential harms (significant risk of *low* blood pressure, fainting and deterioration in kidney function). Lifestyle measures (diet, exercise, weight loss) had not been tried before putting participants on medication. The multiple medications needed to achieve the 120 target in most participants would bring all the well-known dangers of polypharmacy. Since 90 people needed to be treated to prevent one death, 89 in every 90 would be treated unnecessarily. A previous Cochrane review of comparable (although not identical) studies found no benefit in reducing systolic blood pressure below 140 mmHg [3]. Some statisticians questioned the justification for stopping the trial early. And so on.

As our colleagues in the humanities are fond of telling us, there is no text that is self-interpreting. That maxim applies as much to a randomised controlled trial as to Shakespeare's plays. Facts, as I will argue in Section 9.3, are value-laden. The trade-off between risks and benefits for an individual patient is always a matter of judgement and preference. That, of course, is why clinicians need wisdom as well as evidence.

In a recent paper on knowledge mobilisation in complex systems (see Chapter 11 for more on those), Bev Holmes and colleagues said this:

> *The very meaning of evidence is now the subject of lively debate. However defined, the emerging consensus is that evidence is not a thing apart, generated in isolation and then passed on to those who will use it. It is clear that evidence alone does not solve problems, and that myriad elements of context – including different professional, organisational and sectoral cultures and the role of power and politics – are critical considerations.* [4]

In sum, even scientifically 'robust' research evidence has a history and a context. It may be inherently uncertain, incomplete and open to multiple interpretations. It sits better in some contexts than others. And it competes for our attention with many other issues, some of which are extremely important. As we consider the question of how to implement research evidence, let us bear in mind that such evidence is rarely a set of final and incontrovertible 'facts' that simply need to be cascaded into practice. Much of the rest of this book picks up on this central theme.

2.2 Knowledge translation, knowledge transfer

Let us put aside for now the contestability and inherent uncertainty of research evidence, and assume that there *is* a set of research findings that are relevant to the issue at hand. The remainder of this chapter considers how to maximise the chances of that evidence being accessed, understood and put into practice by clinicians, managers, policymakers and patients. In other words, I will be addressing the science, art and practice of *knowledge translation*. Be warned – I base much of this section on an article I co-authored a few years ago entitled 'Is it Time to Drop the Knowledge Translation Metaphor?' [5].

'Knowledge translation' is a relatively new term that has come to replace the older concept of *knowledge transfer,* used to depict the one-way shift of research knowledge from researchers to – well, just about anyone else. Jonathan Lomas usefully depicted a continuum with three essential processes:

1. diffusion (a passive phenomenon akin to osmosis);
2. dissemination (involving active efforts from researchers and intermediaries to raise awareness and promote interest in research findings);
3. implementation (involving proactive efforts to understand the needs of the research user and follow-through to achieve a change in behaviour) [6].

In today's terminology, the first two processes might be considered knowledge transfer; the third, knowledge translation.

Knowledge translation was originally defined at a consensus meeting of the World Health Organization (WHO) in 2005:

> *the synthesis, exchange and application of knowledge by relevant stakeholders to accelerate the benefits of global and local innovation in strengthening health systems and advancing people's health.* [7]

More recently, this definition was refined by the Canadian Institutes of Health Research (CIHR):

> *a dynamic and iterative process that includes the synthesis, dissemination, exchange and ethically sound application of knowledge to improve health, provide more effective health services and products and strengthen the healthcare system.* [8]

At the original WHO consensus meeting in 2005, successful knowledge translation was conceptualised as dependent on 'supply' or 'push factors' (availability of evidence; appropriate packaging, e.g. in 'evidence-based actionable messages'; credible knowledge brokers and opinion leaders) and 'demand' or 'pull factors' (e.g. local knowledge champions; political support for implementation of particular research evidence; strategic presence on local decision-making bodies). Barriers to knowledge translation were likewise divided into push factors (e.g. evidence too complex; cost of producing, packaging and distributing evidence too prohibitive; poor local access to relevant evidence) and pull factors (e.g. low demand for scientific evidence by policymakers; political and/or financial reasons for not acting on evidence; 'paradigm differences' between researchers, policymakers and practitioners) [7].

Many published analyses of the knowledge translation challenge offer similar taxonomies of problems and solutions. Clinicians, it is lamented, only rarely follow evidence-based guidelines; managers and policymakers fail to draw consistently on robust evidence when designing services or allocating resources (for more on those challenges, see Sections 3.3 and 9.1 respectively). Solutions to these problems are generally framed in terms of a more efficient 'evidence pathway', 'evidence-based decision support', 'evidence-based policy-making' and 'evidence-based management' – all of which entail the controlled supply of research evidence that has been vetted, summarised and made accessible to its intended audience and/or the shaping of demand for this evidence through education, facilitation, financial incentives or inscription of decision pathways into technology.

Three assumptions underpin the knowledge translation metaphor. The first is that 'knowledge' equates with objective, impersonal research findings – a form of what Aristotle called *episteme* and later writers have called *explicit knowledge* (for more on explicit versus tacit knowledge, see Section 10.1). In basic science, research evidence means consistent and reproducible laboratory findings; in health services research, it means (usually) randomised controlled trials or meta-analyses; in management, it may mean findings from cognitive psychology about how people assimilate information or what motivates them. In all these cases, knowledge is seen as unproblematically separable from the scientists who generate it and the practitioners who may use it (the 'objectivist' approach to knowledge).

The second assumption is that it is useful to conceptualise a 'know–do gap' between scientific facts and practice (whether in the clinical encounter, in the management of staff or around the policymaking table). This implies that knowledge and practice can be cleanly separated, both empirically and analytically.

The third assumption is that practice consists more or less of a series of rational decisions on which scientific research findings can be brought to bear.

These three assumptions are widely held within the medical field, but as Sietse Wieringa and I argued in our paper [5], and as I argue in more depth in the remainder of this book, they are widely questioned by scholars outside it.

In brief, knowledge is not so easily separated from the context in which it was generated (or the context in which it has been successfully applied); transferring successful innovations or service models from setting A to setting B is notoriously difficult [9]. The 'know–do gap' is appealing in its simplicity, but filling gaps may turn out to be a misleading metaphor in the social science of improving practice. Neither clinical practice nor policy-making is, in reality, an exercise in rational decision science.

Despite these caveats, the metaphor of knowledge translation is neither obsolete nor useless – so long as you remember that it is something of an oversimplification. It can apply pretty well in some contexts – but falls very flat in others (see Section 10.1 for more detail on such contexts). In the last Section (2.5), I offer tips for improving your knowledge translation skills.

2.3 Different worlds

If you inhabit the world of research, there is nothing more robust, nothing more meaningful and nothing more exciting than a well-conducted empirical study or systematic review that has been written up in IMRaD (Introduction, Methods, Results and Discussion) format and published in an academic journal. You may or may not be aware that not everyone inhabits your world. But to convey your research knowledge effectively, you must reflect on the assumptions and priorities of your own world and learn about the very different worlds of non-researchers.

In the world of research, we value precision, accuracy, logical argument, careful measurement and detailed analysis. Getting an answer correct, and perhaps checking it using more than one set of instruments, is viewed as more important than producing an answer by a certain date or keeping a study within an allocated budget. Research involves questioning, challenging and attempting to replicate (or, indeed, refute) the work of other researchers. Its goal is usually to produce generalisable findings, free of the ephemera of any particular context.

Given these priorities, it is not surprising that the research world is oriented to producing lengthy, pedantic, jargon-ridden papers that address narrowly defined questions and which centre on abstract variables whilst systematically and carefully excluding (or 'controlling for') any local, here-and-now contingencies.

In the clinical world, excellence is defined differently. Good clinical practice draws on objective science (including examining the patient, selecting and interpreting tests and finding and applying relevant research evidence), but it also involves contextual judgement and attention to the subjective experience of the particular patient being treated. Above all else, the clinician asks an ethical and uniquely personal question: What is the right thing to do, for *this* patient in *this* situation, *today*? This may include asking whether the patient and the healthcare system can afford the tests or treatments on offer, and whether allocating a particular investigation or treatment to the patient might create a shortfall elsewhere in the system.

For all these reasons, and as John Ioannidis recently argued, research is very often not actually *useful* to clinicians [10]. A clinically useful research study satisfies the criteria listed in Box 2.1.

I live in hope that the next generation of clinical research will pay more attention to usefulness than the previous generation(s). But right now, the mismatch between what researchers produce and what clinicians want and need can be almost comical.

As I will explain in more detail in Chapter 9, the policy world sings in yet another key [11]. Policymaking is about defining and pursuing the right course of action in a particular context, at a particular time, for a particular group of people and with a particular allocation of resources. Policymaking requires decisions to be timely and to fit with the (usually annual) cycle of

---

Box 2.1 What is a clinically useful research study?

A clinically useful research study satisfies the following criteria:

- It was designed to address a real and important problem (as opposed to focusing on one that has been concocted by disease mongerers or intervention zealots, for example).
- It adds substantially and systematically to what we already know (i.e. its authors began with a thorough review of the literature, identified a key knowledge gap and set out to fill it).
- Its design was pragmatic (i.e. the study participants and context reflect real-world patients and circumstances rather than a highly selected 'clean' patient sample who are given extra attention and fringe benefits).
- It measured outcomes that matter to patients (rather than blood test results, blobs on X-rays or other surrogate endpoints).
- The intervention is good value for money (hence, if it 'works', healthcare funders will be able to afford it without axing some other crucial service).
- The intervention is feasible and acceptable in the real world.
- The study data are available for verification and challenge (as opposed to locked up in a 'commercial-in-confidence' file kept by company lawyers – in which case most people won't trust the findings).

Source: Adapted from Ioannidis [10].

resource allocation. Getting *something* on the table for next Monday's board meeting is often more important than waiting for researchers to finish analysing their data. And the only evidence policymakers currently want is evidence to address the problems they have defined as the current priorities. Finally, whilst many (although not all) researchers are still focused exclusively on randomised controlled trial evidence, because someone told them it was the 'gold standard', policymakers actually need a much wider range of evidence, including broad-ranging 'scoping reviews' of key topic areas, qualitative studies, economic evaluations and policy analyses [12].

Whilst we are exploring the worlds of non-researchers, spare a thought for the patient. As I wrote with some colleagues in a paper recently:

> *Even when patients are 'informed', 'empowered', and 'health-literate' (and especially when they are not), they rarely inhabit a world of controlled experiments, abstracted variables, objective measurement of pre-defined outcomes, average results, or generalizable truths. Rather, they live in the messy, idiosyncratic, and unpredictable world of a particular person in a particular family context (or, for some, in a context of social isolation and/or abandonment by family) … The clinical encounter, whether patient-initiated (e.g. to present a symptom or concern) or clinician-initiated (e.g. an invitation for screening or chronic disease surveillance), has cultural and moral significance and occurs against a complex backdrop of personal sense making, information seeking, and lay consultations.* [13]

I will pick up on the 'worlds' of clinicians, policymakers and patients in later chapters, but for now, let us just recognise that the conventional outputs of the scientific research community are not usually the right size or shape, nor are they produced to the right timescale, to meet the needs of any of these groups [14]. The tips for knowledge translation in Section 2.5 are designed to better align the outputs of academic research with the needs of people who use (or might use) such research.

2.4 Attributes of innovations

Diffusion of innovation theory was developed in relation to individual adopters by Everett Rogers [15] and extended by my own team to encompass the organisational and system context of healthcare innovation (see Chapter 5) [16]. Rogers defined an innovation as 'an idea, practice or object that is perceived as new'. He certainly included research evidence within that definition (he was a social scientist studying the adoption by American farmers of new farming practices developed by university researchers).

> **Box 2.2 Attributes of innovations**
>
> An innovation is an idea, practice or object that is perceived as new. An innovation is more likely to be adopted if potential adopters consider that it has the following attributes:
>
> - **Relative advantage:** The innovation is better or more efficient than whatever is currently used.
> - **Low complexity:** The innovation is simple to understand and use (or, if complex, can be broken down into simpler components).
> - **Compatibility:** The innovation and its use align with prevailing values and ways of working.
> - **Observability:** The effects of the innovation are easily observed and measured, and can be unambiguously attributed to it.
> - **Trialability:** The innovation can be tried out on a small scale before people commit.
> - **Potential for reinvention:** Users can customise the innovation to suit personal preferences and/or local circumstances.
> - **Ease of use (for technologies):** The innovation is easy to use and/or comes with adequate technical support.
>
> *Source: Adapted from Rogers* [15].

Summarising his own research and that of others, Rogers identified a number of features ('attributes' as perceived by potential adopters) of innovations that tend to promote their adoption in practice. These are listed in Box 2.2.

Of all the attributes in Box 2.2, the single most important – for research evidence, as for almost all other innovations – is *relative advantage*. If a clinician does not believe that following the recommendations from the SPRINT trial would be in the best interests of eligible patients, or believes that following these recommendations would be practically possible, he or she will almost certainly not even attempt to follow them. Conversely, if the clinician *is* convinced that SPRINT represents a new and achievable gold standard of care for people at high risk of cardiovascular events, practice is very likely to change.

I cannot stress this point enough. Far too many papers and books about implementing evidence place too much emphasis on minor details and not enough on the central issue on which the adoption decision turns: *Is the clinician (or manager, or policymaker, or patient) persuaded by the evidence and does he or she believe that change is possible?*

Many of the other attributes in Rogers' original list (e.g. compatibility, observability and trialability) and in the numerous lists of attributes that have been demonstrated in empirical studies of guideline adoption are, to a large extent, factors that explain whether potential adopters are likely to be *persuaded by the evidence* and whether they believe the recommendations will be *workable in practice*.

Incidentally, if you are hungry for more attributes, try Richard Shiffman's 10-point list: decidability, executability, general characteristics, presentation and formatting, measurable outcomes, apparent validity, flexibility, effect on process of care, novelty and computability [17], or even Anna Gagliardi's 22-attribute list for guideline implementablity, grouped under adaptability, usability, validity, applicability, communicability, accommodation, implementation and evaluation [18]. Personally, I find relative advantage, low complexity and trialability cover most bases when I am asking questions about innovations.

The importance of relative advantage (the intended adopter's belief that the innovation represents a new standard of best practice) has been shown empirically in numerous studies. In an early study of guideline adoption, for example, Richard Grol's team in the Netherlands showed that the attributes of clinical guidelines most strongly associated with their being followed were (i) whether they were 'controversial' (i.e. whether the clinicians disagreed with the recommendation – if they did, they rarely followed it); (ii) whether the instructions were clear and specific; and (iii) whether the guidelines demanded a change in practice (if they did, they were less likely to be followed). Complexity had a statistically significant but small influence on the overall impact of a guideline (in other words, if clinicians believed the evidence for a change in practice was strong, the complexity of new recommendations rarely held them back).

Other empirical studies have shown similar findings. I discuss Grol's study in more depth in Section 3.4, when I talk about approaches to changing clinicians' perspectives on guidelines with a view to influencing their behaviour.

2.5 Ten tips for translating evidence

In this section, I have assumed that you are a researcher who has produced some new findings in the form of an academic report or guideline. However, these tips work equally well if you are a change agent who is seeking to translate some evidence you have found in the existing literature. I have drawn on an extensive evidence base on what works in knowledge translation [5,12,18–24].

1. Shorten

Evidence-based guidelines might (at best) provide a counsel of perfection, but the volume of evidence now available is widely recognised to be unmanageable. In one study, the guidelines relevant to investigating and treating 18 patients admitted by one medical team over 24 hours ran to 3679 pages [25].

Similarly, a recent paper entitled 'What Makes an Academic Paper Useful for Health Policy?' pointed out that policymakers are both busy and swamped with evidence, and that by far the most useful paper an academic can produce is a rigorous and succinct summary of *all* the evidence on a topic [12].

The art of *shortening* a research publication includes (but is certainly not limited to):

- Editing down a 5000-word paper to 2500 words (far too many scientific papers are lazily written and unnecessarily verbose – and many Nobel prizes have been won on papers only two or three pages long).
- Putting particular effort into crafting the abstract (this is the only part most people will ever read).
- Using the 1-3-25 format for reports (25 pages maximum for the main text, with any additional material shifted into appendices; a 3-page executive summary designed for the non-academic reader that makes sense without the need to refer to the main text; and a 1-page covering letter or press release listing the key findings and implications as bullet points).
- Developing an 'elevator pitch' of the three most important findings from the study.
- Turning the findings into a 140-charater message for Twitter (see Tip 9).

2. Sharpen

Merely shortening your research message will not necessarily make it accessible to potential users. You need to think carefully about which aspects to omit and which to bring to the surface in your summary. Potential users of research evidence do not want oversimplification. Indeed, a piece of evidence is more likely to be taken up and to influence practice if it sets out the strength and quality of evidence and the current state of knowledge (What do we know?), but also the state of ignorance (What don't we know?) and uncertainty (On which points is there residual disagreement or inherent ambiguity?).

As a rule of thumb, your summary should include one sentence of background (Why does this matter? Why now?), one sentence on the study design and methods (What did you do, and how?), two sentences on the key findings (What did you find?) and one or two sentences providing a conclusion and discussing the implications (What do you think should change as a result of your research?). Many journals ask for a 'structured abstract' in which each of these sections has its own subheading.

This sounds straightforward but is actually a difficult task (recall the apocryphal story of Blaise Pascal's covering note: 'I'm sorry to send a long letter; I didn't have time to write a short one'). Remember that on the one hand the non-academic reader may be more interested in the potential implications of your findings than in the detail of the findings themselves, but on the other researchers are notoriously bad at judging what the policy implications of their work are (because whilst they understand the research dimension, they do not understand the complex nature of the policy process) – a point I pick up in Section 9.4.

3. Tailor

A fundamental principle of marketing is that different audiences have different needs, learning styles, preferences and so on [15]. It follows that the overall target audience for a research message needs to be *segmented*, and the message carefully tailored to the different segments (i.e. subgroups). The same set of research findings will need to be presented differently (i.e. 'framed') to make it maximally appealing to fellow academics (and within that group, members of one's own discipline will need a different message from those in other disciplines), clinicians (nurses, doctors, allied professionals, students and so on), policymakers (national, local), managers (top, middle), finance directors, citizens (taxpayers, voters), the media (specialist or generalist, broadsheet or tabloid) and potential patients (from different cultural backgrounds and with varying degrees of health literacy).

To tailor your message, ideally you should do some 'market audience research' (interviews, focus groups, surveys) to find out:

- What each target group already knows and believes about the topic.
- What their relevant assumptions and values are.
- What rumours, myths and misinformation exist about the topic in this community.
- What information people would like, and what they identify as their knowledge gaps.

In practice, formal research to inform the tailoring of messages is rarely undertaken (perhaps more of it should be funded), but you may gain useful information from an analysis of published literature and/or discussions with people who have dealt with similar audiences previously.

4. Narrativise

Get this: your research is almost certainly boring. Hence, there is a high chance that your audience may lose interest before it reaches the end of your account. Telling stories is a time-honoured way of making boring topics more interesting.

Aristotle suggested that a story (narrative) has five key characteristics: a setting; an unfolding of events and actions over time; characters (people to whom these events and actions happen); emplotment (the rhetorical juxtaposition of the characters, events and actions to evoke meaning, motive and causality); and trouble (peripeteia – the unexpected in the form of surprise, a 'twist in the plot' and so on). A story takes dry, abstract findings and humanises them.

In a blog entitled 'Once Upon a Time in Marketingland…', I found the following advice on the use of stories in marketing a product [26]:

- *Storytelling is a proven way to develop identity, build your client base, and increase sales.*
- *Stories immediately focus on engagement, experiences, and emotion – central tenets that are catnip to customers.*
- *Narrative makes your message relevant and memorable through personalisation.*
- *Through narrative, you can create campaigns to challenge the big players, even on the most thrifty of budgets.*
- *Storytelling conveys to customers, the media, and investors the information, hard facts, and dry data they need in an easily digestible way.*
- *Creative narrative is guaranteed to get people's attention and keep your business front of mind.*

These recommendations were designed, no doubt, to sell refrigerators or sausages, but they are equally pertinent to the marketing of research findings.

The value of narrative in knowledge translation has been demonstrated in randomised controlled trials. For example, Paul Shekelle's team showed that physicians who received guidelines on electrodiagnostic tests (EDTs) for patients with low back pain were more likely to use them appropriately if the guidelines included vignettes illustrating their use in patients with differing indications than if they did not [27]. Similarly, health education in which the message is framed as a story may be more effective than education given as 'facts' [28,29]. One group of researchers has even developed a 'narrative engagement framework' for designing preventive interventions [30].

5. Visualise

What do people do when flicking through a report or walking through a poster exhibition? Most pick out the visuals and read only the associated captions (10-word summaries of what each image shows). This is not such a bad tactic. Visuals (graphs, maps, diagrams and so on) can achieve a great deal in a small space [31].

Good visuals display data efficiently and in a way that highlights rather than distorts key findings; they encourage comparison between selected pieces of data; and they prevent distraction by other parts of the dataset.

Visuals can present data at multiple levels (e.g. they can 'zoom out' to give a coherent overview and 'zoom in' to finer structure). As John Berger illustrates brilliantly in his book *Ways of Seeing*, because the creation of a graph, image, or map involves the selective highlighting of some data at the expense of others, a visual is an excellent way of framing an issue in a particular way (see Tip 3) [32]. It follows that different target audiences may need different visuals.

People gather round visuals and argue about them. Like stories, pictures are evocative and demand an explanation. They prompt conversations about what the data *mean* and what should be *done*.

Figure 2.1, reproduced from Public Health England Obesity (PHE Obesity; a national data archive of overweight and obesity levels over time), includes 80 data points (along with confidence intervals) from the National Child Measurement Programme (NCMP). It depicts two important trends (increase in child obesity with increasing socio-economic deprivation and increase in child obesity over time) and an interaction between the two: the more deprived the subgroup, the greater the increase in obesity level over time (indeed, for the most affluent subgroups, obesity levels have begun to reduce over time).

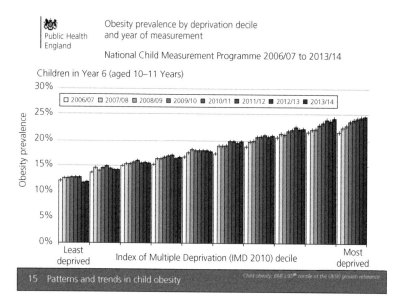

Figure 2.1   Visual display of child weight data by deprivation index, 2006/07–2013/14. *Source*: Public Health England (http://www.noo.org.uk/NOO_pub/Key_data, accessed October 2016).

All this prompts (but does not answer) questions such as 'What is causing these trends?', 'To what extent is this a public health problem?' and 'What should we do about it?'. My purpose in including this visual in this chapter was not, of course, to answer these questions, but to illustrate how pictures get people engaged and asking questions.

6. Recruit key messengers

Aristotle, who has already featured in this list once in relation to narrative, also introduced the memorable triad of what is needed in order for evidence to have an impact:

- *logos* (the evidence itself, the 'facts' of a case);
- *ethos* (the credibility of the speaker or writer who conveys those facts);
- *pathos* (the appeal to emotions – an aspect of tailoring or framing) [33].

Aristotle's insight was that facts, whatever their importance, are rarely taken up without the personal intervention of someone who has credibility with their potential audience(s). Different audiences will assign a different level of *ethos* to different people.

There is much empirical evidence that persuasion to change behaviour in line with an evidence-based recommendation generally requires inter-personal communication from an individual known to the potential adopter of the recommendation. Those who undertake such persuasion work go by a lot of different names (opinion leaders, champions, change agents and so on). I cover them in detail in Section 10.2.

7. Mobilise the media

Whilst individual, interpersonal input is generally needed to persuade some-one to change, mass media can play an important role in *creating awareness* of something that might be changed [15]. Mass media can be generalist (e.g. national newspapers, TV and the Internet equivalent) or specialist (the so-called 'grey literature' of non-academic publications aimed at clin-icians, policymakers and so on). Don't forget that specialists also read generalist literature, so an excellent way of alerting (say) doctors to a new research finding is to get a story into a national newspaper.

Some of the worst literature I have ever read in my life consists of so-called press releases written by academics. The world of research is a million miles away from the world of journalism (especially tabloid journalism), and researchers often make a boring study even more boring when they try to popularise it. Box 2.3 gives some tips for writing scientific press releases, adapted (curiously enough) from a section of the website for the Hubble Space Telescope.

> **Box 2.3 Tips for writing scientific press releases**
>
> 1 **Hot or not?:** Is there a newsworthy angle to your announcement (e.g. has something new and important happened; does it have local or national relevance; has the discovery settled an ongoing controversy; is there a human interest angle)?
>
> 2 **Get expert help:** You may be terrible at writing press releases, but your university probably has a communications ('press') office where much talent may be found.
>
> 3 **Participate in shaping the message:** Preparing a press release takes time and effort. Be prepared to spend time explaining the science and extracting key information for the communications expert.
>
> 4 **Involve other institutions:** If you have collaborated with other research groups, link the different communications offices and work with them on a joint press release, ideally aiming for simultaneous co-release.
>
> 5 **Create images:** An appropriate image or illustration helps sell your message, but images taken from 'stock' can be misleading or deadening. Work with your communications office to create appealing and correct imagery.
>
> 6 **Add value:** Your press release will have far greater impact if you back it up with a more specialised web page containing additional information (e.g. links to your academic outputs, translations of the press release into other languages, additional images, graphs, a video).
>
> Source: *Adapted from* www.spacetelescope.org. *Accessed October 2016. Reproduced with permission of ESO.*

8. Blog

'Blog' is short for 'web log' – in other words, an account you write yourself and upload on to the World Wide Web. The technical aspects are not difficult. Try putting 'How to start a blog' into Google and then follow the step-by-step guides to getting yourself a domain (a place on the World Wide Web to site your writing), choosing a catchy name for your blog, designing an attractive layout, uploading text and adding pictures and hyperlinks (links to other sites on the Web). More difficult is getting the writing style right. With no explicit word count, you may find yourself rambling, and the informal nature of blogs makes it easy to slip into a vernacular style that some readers will find irritating and unprofessional.

Perhaps the best way to start blogging is to read other people's blogs and pick up on a style you like. My favourite bloggers include Richard Lehman, who writes a weekly review of medical journals (http://blogs.bmj.com/bmj/category/richard-lehmans-weekly-review-of-medical-journals/); Disruptive

Women in Healthcare (well I would, wouldn't I? http://www.disruptivewomen.net/blog/); and KevinMD (http://www.kevinmd.com/blog/). All are engaging, upbeat, varied and funny, and all cover important topics.

My own tips on writing blogs are:

a. Don't just write. Write for a specific audience and try to persuade that audience of something.
b. Make one key point per blog post, keeping your text short (800 words is a good rule of thumb) and using stories and visuals (see Tips 4 and 5).
c. Don't overuse hyperlinks: they are confusing, and you'll lose your readers if you keep sending them to other sites every few lines.

9. Tweet

Social media, which might be viewed as a combination of mass media (in that it can reach large numbers) and interpersonal communication (in that people generally choose to link to a specific person) can be a powerful way of reaching certain audiences. My own favourite site is Twitter. Figure 2.2 shows a tweet I sent out about a splendid paper I found that offered a new theoretical perspective on what might be called bad habits (smoking, drinking and so on) [34]. The tweet included a link to the paper so people could check it out for themselves. Many people who saw my tweet liked the paper too, and after only a few hours, my message had been retweeted more than 30 times. Since each tweeter had between 100 and 20 000 followers, my original 140-character message reached many thousands of people, all of whom had previously chosen to follow me or one of my followers (and hence, would be more likely than a randomly mailed person to find this material interesting).

Trisha Greenhalgh @trishgreenhalgh · Dec 21
Unhealthy habits as social practices.
Important challenge to the 'individual behaviour' frame that dominates policy.
tandfonline.com/doi/abs/10.108...

RETWEETS   LIKES
31   32

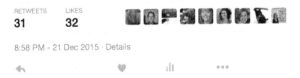

8:58 PM - 21 Dec 2015 · Details

Figure 2.2   Example of tweeting a link to a research paper.

Research on the use of social media to disseminate research findings is in its infancy. I cite little of it here because I am unimpressed with its quality, although I recommend Lutz Bornmann's review of 'altmetrics' (alternative metrics – including 'retweets' on Twitter, 'likes' on Facebook and similar) [35] and a more recent review of the wider science of 'scientometrics' [36].

10. Bundle

Busy clinicians are not usually opposed in principle to doing things that are evidence-based, but they do have multiple competing priorities. If you can align a set of evidence-based recommendations into a 'bundle' of care that gets implemented via a single checklist that is part of business as usual, you will increase the chance of each and all of the items being implemented. A paper by Laura Lennox illustrates how it's done [37], and in Appendix A I offer some practical tips on how to develop a care bundle.

References

1. Ioannidis, J.P. (2005). Why most published research findings are false. *Chance*, **18**(4), 40–47.
2. Wright, J.T. Jr., Williamson, J.D., Whelton, P.K., Snyder, J.K., Sink, K.M., Rocco, M.V., et al. (2015). A randomized trial of intensive versus standard blood-pressure control. *The New England Journal of Medicine*, **373**(22), 2103–2116.
3. Musini, V.M., Tejani, A.M., Bassett, K., & Wright, J.M. (2009). Pharmacotherapy for hypertension in the elderly. *The Cochrane Library*, 7;(4):CD000028.
4. Holmes, B.J., Best, A., Davies, H., Hunter, D., Kelly, M.P., Marshall, M., & Rycroft-Malone, J. (2016). Mobilising knowledge in complex health systems: a call to action. *Evidence & Policy*, https://doi.org/10.1332/174426416X14712553750311.
5. Greenhalgh, T., & Wieringa, S. (2011). Is it time to drop the 'knowledge translation' metaphor? A critical literature review. *Journal of the Royal Society of Medicine*, **104**(12), 501–509.
6. Lomas, J. (1993). Diffusion, dissemination, and implementation: who should do what? *Annals of the New York Academy of Sciences*, **703**(1), 226–237.
7. World Health Organisation (2005). Bridging the 'Know–Do' gap: Meeting on knowledge translation in global health 10–12 October 2005. Geneva, WHO. Available from: https://web.archive.org/web/20110703085501/http://www.who.int/kms/KTGH%20meeting%20report,%20Oct'05.pdf (last accessed 14 January 2017).
8. Straus, S.E., Tetroe, J., & Graham, I. (2009). Defining knowledge translation. *Canadian Medical Association Journal*, **181**(3–4), 165–168.
9. Greenhalgh, T., Robert, G., Bate, P., Kyriakidou, O., & Macfarlane, F. (2005). *Diffusion of Innovations in Health Service Organisations: A Systematic Literature Review*. Oxford, Blackwell.
10. Ioannidis, J.P. (2016). Why most clinical research is not useful. *PLoS Medicine*, **13**(6), e1002049.

11. Greenhalgh, T., & Russell, J. (2009). Evidence-based policymaking: a critique. *Perspectives in Biology and Medicine*, **52**(2), 304–318.
12. Whitty, C.J. (2015). What makes an academic paper useful for health policy? *BMC Medicine*, **13**(1), 1.
13. Greenhalgh, T., Snow, R., Ryan, S., Rees, S., & Salisbury, H. (2015). Six 'biases' against patients and carers in evidence-based medicine. *BMC Medicine*, **13**(1), 200.
14. George, A.L. (1994). The two cultures of academia and policy-making: bridging the gap. *Political Psychology*, **15**(1), 143–172.
15. Rogers, E.M. (2010). *Diffusion of Innovations*, 5th edn. London, Simon and Schuster.
16. Greenhalgh, T., Robert, G., Macfarlane, F., Bate, P., & Kyriakidou, O. (2004). Diffusion of innovations in service organizations: systematic review and recommendations. *The Milbank Quarterly*, **82**(4), 581–629.
17. Shiffman, R.N., Dixon, J., Brandt, C., Essaihi, A., Hsiao, A., Michel, G., & O'Connell, R. (2005). The GuideLine Implementability Appraisal (GLIA): development of an instrument to identify obstacles to guideline implementation. *BMC Medical Informatics and Decision Making*, **5**(1), 23.
18. Gagliardi, A.R., Brouwers, M.C., Palda, V.A., Lemieux-Charles, L., & Grimshaw, J.M. (2011). How can we improve guideline use? A conceptual framework of implementability. *Implementation Science*, **6**(1), 26.
19. Oliver, K., Innvar, S., Lorenc, T., Woodman, J., & Thomas, J. (2014). A systematic review of barriers to and facilitators of the use of evidence by policymakers. *BMC Health Services Research*, **14**(1), 2.
20. Eccles, M.P., Armstrong, D., Baker, R., Cleary, K., Davies, H., Davies, S., et al. (2009). An implementation research agenda. *Implementation Science*, **4**(1), 18.
21. Graham, K.E.R., Chorzempa, H.L., Valentine, P.A., & Magnan, J. (2012). Evaluating health research impact: development and implementation of the Alberta Innovates – Health Solutions impact framework. *Research Evaluation*, **21**(5), 354–367.
22. Long, J.C., Cunningham, F.C., & Braithwaite, J. (2013). Bridges, brokers and boundary spanners in collaborative networks: a systematic review. *BMC Health Services Research*, **13**(1), 158.
23. McCormack, L., Sheridan, S., Lewis, M., Boudewyns, V., Melvin, C.L., Kistler, C., et al. (2013). *Communication and Dissemination Strategies to Facilitate the Use of Health-Related Evidence. Evidence Reports/Technology Assessments, No. 213*. Rockville, MD, US Agency for Healthcare Quality.
24. Bero, L.A., Grilli, R., Grimshaw, J.M., Harvey, E., Oxman, A.D., & Thomson, M.A. (1998). Closing the gap between research and practice: an overview of systematic reviews of interventions to promote the implementation of research findings. *BMJ*, **317**(7156), 465–468.
25. Allen, D., & Harkins, K. (2005). Too much guidance? *Lancet*, **365**(9473), 1768.
26. Kissmetrics (2013). Once upon a time in marketingland…why narrative is key to customer engagement. Available from: https://blog.kissmetrics.com/narrative-and-customer-engagement/(last accessed 14 January 2017).

Chapter 2

27. Shekelle, P.G., Kravitz, R.L., Beart, J., Marger, M., Wang, M., & Lee, M. (2000). Are nonspecific practice guidelines potentially harmful? A randomized comparison of the effect of nonspecific versus specific guidelines on physician decision making. *Health Services Research*, **34**(7), 1429–1448.

28. Prati, G., Pietrantoni, L., & Zani, B. (2012). Influenza vaccination: the persuasiveness of messages among people aged 65 years and older. *Health Communication*, **27**(5), 413–420.

29. Murphy, S.T., Frank, L.B., Chatterjee, J.S., Moran, M.B., Zhao, N., Amezola de Herrera, P., & Baezconde-Garbanati, L.A. (2015). Comparing the relative efficacy of narrative vs nonnarrative health messages in reducing health disparities using a randomized trial. *American Journal of Public Health*, **105**(10), 2117–2123.

30. Miller-Day, M., & Hecht, M.L. (2013). Narrative means to preventative ends: a narrative engagement framework for designing prevention interventions. *Health Communication*, **28**(7), 657–670.

31. Tufte, E.R., & Graves-Morris, P. (1983). *The Visual Display of Quantitative Information*, Vol. **2**. Cheshire, CT, Graphics Press.

32. Berger, J. (2008). *Ways of Seeing*, Vol. **1**. London, Penguin.

33. Aristotle [1991]. *The Art of Rhetoric*, trans. Hugh Lawson-Tancred. Harmondsworth, Penguin.

34. Blue, S., Shove, E., Carmona, C., & Kelly, M.P. (2016). Theories of practice and public health: understanding (un) healthy practices. *Critical Public Health*, **26**(1), 36–50.

35. Bornmann, L. (2014). Do altmetrics point to the broader impact of research? An overview of benefits and disadvantages of altmetrics. *Journal of Informetrics*, **8**(4), 895–903.

36. Mingers, J., & Leydesdorff, L. (2015). A review of theory and practice in scientometrics. *European Journal of Operational Research*, **246**(1), 1–19.

37. Lennox, L., Green, S., Howe, C., Musgrave, H., Bell, D., & Elkin, S. (2014). Identifying the challenges and facilitators of implementing a COPD care bundle. *BMJ Open Respiratory Research*, **1**(1), e000035.

Chapter 3 **People**

3.1 Introduction

A few years ago, in our systematic review of the diffusion of innovations in healthcare organisations [1], my team drew the following conclusion about people:

People are not passive recipients of innovations. Rather (and to a greater or lesser extent in different persons), they seek innovations, experiment with them, evaluate them, find (or fail to find) meaning in them, develop feelings (positive or negative) about them, challenge them, worry about them, complain about them, 'work around' them, gain experience with them, modify them to fit particular tasks, and try to improve or redesign them – often through dialogue with other users. (p. 598)

That became the most widely quoted paragraph I've ever written.

In my opinion, far too much research on changing clinical practice uses the same stimulus–response language and methods that psychologists have used to study the behaviour of animals (the very fact that researchers tend to use the term 'behaviour' in relation to professional practice, for example, is telling). The assumption seems to be that we adopt and sustain behaviours for which we are rewarded and abandon behaviours for which we are punished. (Behaviourism's roots include the work of Ivan Pavlov, who undertook studies of classical conditioning in dogs in the 1890s and of B.F. Skinner, who extended this approach to both animals and humans in the mid 20th century [2]. Skinner's work on operant conditioning in rats showed that the more a rat was rewarded for a behaviour, the more it exhibited that behaviour. The same was often true of humans – under laboratory conditions, at least).

Whilst research into 'incentives' and the like is not necessarily flawed, I believe that people are fundamentally different from animals. They are

How to Implement Evidence-Based Healthcare, First Edition. Trisha Greenhalgh.
© 2018 John Wiley & Sons Ltd. Published 2018 by John Wiley & Sons Ltd.

social and moral beings. They have personalities, values, identities, desires, goals, allegiances and commitments. They care about things – and about people, issues and principles. They imagine. They make and use tools. They plan. They reason. They seek to make sense of their world.

For all these reasons, I believe we will never be able to explain or predict human behaviour using crude stimulus–response models. Rather, we need to *theorise* human behaviour (i.e. carefully and systematically seek to explain what is happening and why) in terms of its underlying drivers, including the social context in which the human contemplates what to do and starts to act. And we need to test our theories empirically in rich, qualitative studies. *Why is person X doing (or refusing to do) Y in context Z?*

Whilst our systematic review of the diffusion of innovations included an important statement about the importance of studying human behaviour in context [1], we did not have the time or resources to explore this phenomenon fully. But we did flag the extensive literature on human psychology as needing a good sort-out. A number of people (including Gerd Gigerenzer, Richard Grol, Jeremy Grimshaw, Susan Michie and – most recently – my own doctoral student, Nick Fahy) have been working on that task for several years. This chapter presents a still-incomplete summary of the key findings in a field that remains hotly contested and extensively researched.

3.2 Theories of human behaviour – an eclectic selection

It is easy to reach saturation on behaviour change theories (later in this chapter, I will tell you there are dozens). I don't know all of them myself, nor do I ever intend to learn them. The theories in this section are the ones I find useful both in my own research and in my efforts to effect change in clinical practice.

'Fast' and 'slow' thinking; heuristics; cognitive biases (Kahneman, Gigerenzer)

In his book, *Thinking, Fast and Slow* (which won him the Nobel Prize for Economic Science in 2002), Daniel Kahneman explored two different kinds of thinking, which he called 'System 1' and 'System 2' [3]. System-1-thinking is rapid, intuitive, associative, metaphorical and effortless. It happens unconsciously and cannot be switched off at will. System-2-thinking is slow, deliberate, logical, deductive and effortful, and requires will and intention.

A medical example of System-1-thinking is provided by a picture of a shingles rash along a classic dermatome: any experienced clinician will look at the rash and immediately *know* that it is shingles. An example of System-2-thinking is the sum 624×72, which requires most of us to embark on a laborious exercise in long multiplication. We can do it, but it's not automatic or quick.

Contrary to many people's assumptions, System-1-thinking is what drives our decision-making and behaviour most of the time – and because it is quick, it tends to keep us out of danger. System 2 takes over when we meet new or difficult problems – although this system often gets tired and is easily distracted.

Whilst most of the step-by-step guides to evidence-based medicine (EBM) (including, arguably, the entire guidelines industry) are predicated on a System-2 model of human reasoning, clinical practice is, in reality, largely a System-1 affair. As psychologist Gerd Gigerenzer has shown, there is considerable evidence that when making real-world judgements, ignoring much of the potentially relevant information can improve the accuracy of our decisions [4–6].

Instead of systematically weighing up all the factors in every decision, for example, clinicians tend to make rapid and intuitive judgements based on what Gigerenzer calls 'fast and frugal heuristics' (i.e. simple rules of thumb that tap into System-1-thinking) [5]. Following an evidence-based guideline or protocol requires us to be highly rational (rule-based, deductive, algorithmic and predictive), whereas the use of heuristics involves an entirely different kind of cognitive processing (analogical, abductive, based on subconscious pattern recognition). Unfortunately, as a narrative review of studies of heuristic reasoning in clinical settings a few years ago showed, we still do not know which clinical situations lend themselves better to heuristics versus the algorithmic reasoning of guidelines [7].

Gigerenzer introduced the notion of *bounded rationality*: the idea that because real-world decisions often involve numerous options, outcomes and contextual factors, we unconsciously simplify the problem to make it easier to cope with cognitively [6].

Heuristics is one way we bound our rationality. Cognitive biases may be another. Such biases are ways in which the brain systematically distorts perception (or the processing of perception), leading to decision-making that is less than rational – or, at least, decision-making that *appears* less rational. Arguably, however, many of the cognitive biases listed in Table 3.1 are actually simplification strategies that allow us to think fast when fast thinking is needed. A recent systematic review of cognitive biases in decision-making suggests that the more you look for them, the more you find them [8].

If you have ever tried to memorise the cognitive biases in Table 3.1, along with the dozens more I omitted to list, you will know that there are too many for comfort. I recently came across a wonderful 'cheat sheet' from Buster Benson, from which I have included an extract (Box 3.1). It groups all the biases under four overarching problems and the tendencies our brains use to overcome them. Neat.

Table 3.1 Some cognitive biases that affect clinical decision-making.

Heuristic	Description
Acceptable risk	Some risks (such as lung cancer from smoking) are subjectively viewed as more acceptable than others (such as vaccine damage), even when the probabilities of occurrence are in the other direction. Hazards generally deemed acceptable are familiar, perceived as under the individual's control, have immediate rather than delayed consequences, and are linked to perceived benefits.
Anchoring bias	In the absence of objective probabilities, people judge risk according to a reference point. This may be arbitrary – for example, the status quo or some perception of what is 'normal'.
Availability bias	Events that are easier to recall are judged as more likely to happen. Recall is influenced by recency, strong emotions and anything that increases memorability (such as press coverage and personal experience).
Categorical safety or danger	People may perceive things as either good or bad, irrespective of exposure or context (e.g. 'natural' products may be viewed as inherently safe). This may make them unreceptive to explanations that introduce complexity into the decision (such as balance of benefit and harm).
Framing effect	A glass can be described as 'half empty' or 'half full' – the problem is the same, but it is framed differently. This can have a direct and powerful impact on the decisions of lay people and professionals. Losses often loom larger than gains.
Gambler's fallacy	People tend to think that future probabilities are altered by past events, even when in reality they are unchanged.
Illusory correlation	Prior beliefs and expectations about what correlates with what lead people to perceive correlations that are not in the data.
Normalcy bias	People can be reluctant to plan for, or respond to, a disaster that has never previously occurred.
Personal v. impersonal risk	Those making judgements about others tend to be less risk-averse than those making judgements about themselves.
Probability v. frequency	Poor decision-making is exacerbated by the use of absolute and relative probabilities. Judgement biases are less common when information is presented as frequencies.
Small-number bias	We cannot meaningfully compare very small risks (e.g. of different adverse effects), such as 1 in 20 000 and 1 in 200 000. Expressing harm as relative rather than absolute risk dramatically shifts the subjective benefit–harm balance because the risk of harm seems greater.

Source: Adapted from Greenhalgh et al. [9].

Box 3.1 Extract from Buster Benson's cognitive bias 'cheat sheet'

The vast literature on cognitive biases can be summarised under four main problems:

Problem 1: Too much information.

There is too much information in the world, so our brains filter almost all of it out, leaving what is most likely to be useful to us. As a result:

- We notice things that are already primed in memory or repeated often.
- Bizarre, funny or visually striking things are more memorable.
- We notice when something has changed.
- We are drawn to details that confirm our own existing perspectives.

Problem 2: Not enough meaning.

The world is very confusing, and we need to make sense of it in order to survive. So we look for meaning. As a result:

- We find stories and patterns even in sparse data.
- We fill in gaps in data using (for example) stereotypes, generalities and prior histories.
- We simplify probabilities and numbers to make them easier to think about.
- We make assumptions about what others are thinking.
- We project our current mindset and assumptions on to the past and future.

Problem 3: Need to act fast.

We are constrained by time and information, but we often need to act fast in the face of uncertainty. As a result:

- We favour the immediate, relatable thing in front of us over the delayed and distant.
- We favour options that appear simple or that have more complete information over more complex, ambiguous options.

Problem 4: What should we remember?

We can only afford to retain the bits of information that are most likely to prove useful in the future. We need to make constant bets and trade-offs around what we try to remember and what we forget. As a result:

- We edit and reinforce some memories after the fact.
- We discard specifics to form generalities.
- We reduce events and lists to their key elements.
- We store memories differently based on how they were experienced.

Source: Summarised and adapted with permission from this link (which gives a more complete list of problems and examples of biases): https://betterhumans. coach.me/cognitive-bias-cheat-sheet-55a472476b18#.hadl5jwlz.

Chapter 3

The theory of planned behaviour (Ajzen and Fishbein)

The theory of planned behaviour is one of the most widely cited psychological theories in implementation science [10]. It began life as the theory of reasoned action [11]. Both these theories propose that our voluntary behaviour is a function of the intention to perform the behaviour, which is determined by our attitudes towards the behaviour, subjective norms (i.e. what we think other people will think) and the amount of control we perceive we have over the behaviour, plus the amount of *actual* control we have over the behaviour.

Thus, so the theory goes, if people evaluate a particular suggested behaviour as positive (attitude), and if they think significant others want them to perform the behaviour (subjective norm), this results in a higher intention (motivation) and they are more likely to perform the behaviour, provided that any external constraints to achieving the suggested behaviour are removed.

The theory of planned behaviour has superficial plausibility, but I wonder how much it is simply tautologous (in other words, a circular argument). It seems logical that we behave in a certain way because we intend to behave that way, and that that intention will be stronger if we rate the behaviour highly and think that others rate it highly too. Dozens, if not hundreds of studies have used questionnaire designs to assess clinicians' intention to follow a guideline and confirmed that they are more likely to do so if they feel positively about it and perceive the prevailing norms to be positive (see a study by Kortteisto et al. [12] on hand hygiene guidelines as an example of the genre).

Arguably, such studies, even if done well, end up saying little more than that if people say they are going to do something, and they think it's a good thing to do and believe others think it is a good thing to do, they are more likely to do it, so long as other factors do not stop them. Perhaps more surprising than the ubiquitous finding that this theory explains some human behaviour is the less widely reported finding that it rarely explains all, or even most, human behaviour! For example, a systematic review of 237 independent prospective tests found that this theory accounted for less than 20% of variability in people's health-related behaviour [13]. A systematic review of studies of guideline adherence showed that it fitted the data rather better, but still accounted for only 39% of the variation [14].

My own interpretation of this literature is that it shows that most human behaviour *cannot* be explained simply by invoking rational intention as a product of attitudes and social norms!

What does the theory of planned behaviour overlook? Perhaps most importantly, that we are not always rational beings [15]. We are influenced by unconscious desires, fears and other emotions, by cognitive biases (see previous subsection), by sheer strength of habit and by irrational forces of which we may be partly or wholly conscious (as anyone who has ever broken a diet will attest). We do quite a lot on impulse, rather than because we have planned to behave that way. As already noted, much of our clinical reasoning is 'fast and frugal', based on pattern recognition, not systematic planning. And our beliefs and attitudes may influence our behaviour through subtle pathways without changing our intentions.

Furthermore, as Falko Sniehotta has pointed out, the theory of planned behaviour is a somewhat static theory: it may (imperfectly) explain the influences on behaviour at a given time point, but (in contrast to, say, stages of change theory or social learning theory) it does not explain how behaviour responds to different influences over time – hence, it is not really a theory of behaviour *change* [15].

In sum, the theory of planned behaviour made it into this chapter mainly because so many people treat it as gospel, but I sometimes wonder how many items of clothing this emperor is actually wearing. My advice: if you see a paper based on this theory, ask yourself whether it provides an adequate and compelling explanation of the data or whether any of the other theories listed in this chapter (or found elsewhere) might fit the data better.

Learning domains: knowledge, skills and attitudes (Bloom)

In the 1950s, a group of researchers led by Benjamin Bloom developed a taxonomy of learning domains, which they divided into *cognitive* (knowledge and mental skills), *psychomotor* (skills) and *affective* (attitudes and emotions) [16].

The cognitive domain of Bloom's taxonomy includes the following categories:

- **Knowledge:** The ability to recall data and/or information.
- **Comprehension:** The ability to understand the meaning and significance of what is known.
- **Application:** The ability to utilise an abstraction or to apply knowledge in a new situation.
- **Analysis:** The ability to question and critique the literature, and (for example) to differentiate facts from opinions.
- **Synthesis:** The ability to integrate different elements or concepts in order to form a sound pattern or structure so a new meaning can be established.
- **Evaluation:** The ability to make judgements about the importance of concepts.

The detail of how to ensure that learners successfully gain knowledge, understanding and application, and how to support the development of what are sometimes called the higher-order skills of analysis, synthesis and evaluation, is beyond the scope of this book. But it should be apparent from this brief summary that being able to pass a classroom exam on critical appraisal doesn't mean someone will be confident or competent at finding and applying research evidence in practice. Knowing how to apply the critical appraisal tick-list to a single paper, for example, should not be equated with the ability to sort out the mountain of literature that typically results from a topic search on Medline. Furthermore, education and training must also include measures to ensure that people *care* about the topic and are motivated to do something about it, and exercises to develop specific *skills*.

Adult learning theory (Kolb, Knowles)

David Kolb's theory of adult learning [17], influenced by the American educationist Malcolm Knowles, has informed a stream of research on how to teach clinicians (and others) evidence-based practice. Kolb proposed that adults are motivated to learn; they are self-directed and responsible; and they desire learning to be purposeful, relevant, practical and (perhaps most significantly of all) immediately applicable to their day-to-day work or lives. Adults attending a course are also typically more problem-centred than curriculum-centred (i.e. they generally go on courses in order to learn to solve particular real-world problems, not to acquire particular knowledge or skills).

Kolb (drawing on previous work by Kurt Lewin) proposed that adult learners learn in cycles consisting of four phases that feed into one another:

1. **Concrete experience:** The learner encounters a new experience or situation.
2. **Reflective observation:** The learner contemplates the meaning of the new experience.
3. **Abstract conceptualisation:** Reflection gives rise to a new idea, or a modification of an existing concept or schema.
4. **Active experimentation:** The learner applies the new idea or concept in practice.

My own view is that this adult learning cycle tends to progress much more quickly when people discuss things with fellow team members (see Chapter 4). Figure 3.1 shows my adaptation of the Kolb/Lewin adult learning cycle, incorporating the importance of team discussions. This insight came from me reflecting on Kolb's original diagram alongside my colleague Anita Berlin (a good example of precisely the issue we were seeking to illustrate!).

This cycle informed an important classification of learning styles. This is not the place to go into detail, but the essential point is that some people learn by manipulating abstract concepts; others learn better by hands-on

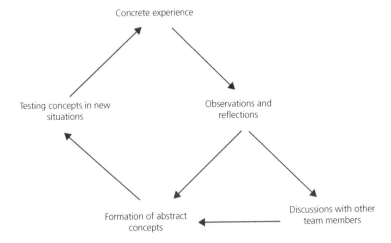

Figure 3.1 The adult learning cycle (adapted to include team discussions).
Source: Elwyn et al. [18] with acknowledgement of an idea from Anita Berlin.

experience; others learn by actively trying to solve problems; and so on. Interventions designed to educate clinicians need to take account of these different learning styles.

Social learning theory and self-efficacy (Bandura)

Social learning theory, originally developed by the social psychologist Albert Bandura in the 1970s [19], is actually a group of theories about learning, all of which are grounded in the belief that human behaviour is determined by a three-way relationship (often depicted as the points of a triangle) between cognitive factors (knowledge, attitudes, expectations), environmental influences (especially social norms) and factors relating to the behaviour (skills, practice, self-efficacy). Some of Bandura's early work on social learning theory was done on children, who seemed to instinctively imitate the behaviour of other children even if they were not encouraged to do so or rewarded for doing so. As the children imitated others, they gained skills and became more confident.

Social learning theory holds that people are more likely to change their behaviour if they:

- observe and imitate the behaviours of others;
- are exposed to positive behaviours modelled and practised;
- increase their own capability and confidence to apply new skills;
- gain positive attitudes about applying these new skills; and
- experience support from their environment in order to use their new skills.

According to this theory, those seeking to change the behaviour of an individual or group of individuals should follow five principles. First, identify role models and provide lots of exposure to these role models. Second, provide hands on training, preferably in groups, so people gain both the necessary knowledge and skills and the confidence to continue exhibiting the new behaviour even when not supervised. Third, ensure that people know about the positive things that will happen if they change their behaviour. Fourth, recognise that there is a reciprocal interaction between the person and the environment (each influencing the other) – getting the best out of the individual may require changing the environment. Fifth, provide incentives and rewards (and encourage self-reward) to reinforce the desired behaviour.

Bandura's work was detailed and rigorous, but his influence on implementation science has been somewhat distorted as non-psychologists have cherry-picked selected elements of his theories and models. One of the most widely adopted aspects of Bandura's work is the construct of self-efficacy, defined as a person's belief in his or her own ability to succeed in specific situations or accomplish a task. Self-efficacy is readily measured using a short questionnaire [20], which means that people doing research on clinician behaviour are often tempted to measure it. Indeed, since measuring clinicians' self-efficacy is a lot easier than measuring what they actually do (or whether this has any impact on patient outcomes), this construct is surprisingly often used as the primary outcome measure in intervention research. I don't dispute that self-efficacy is important, but I don't think Bandura ever intended it to be used as a dipstick to measure the quality of human input to implementing evidence.

So whilst I much prefer social learning theory to the theory of planned behaviour, I feel that too many authors of studies on changing clinician behaviour have taken the line of least resistance and conflated a clinician's score on a self-efficacy scale with whether the intervention to change that clinician's behaviour 'works'. Incidentally, self-efficacy is widely used as an outcome measure in studies of patient self-management education; I cover such studies in Section 7.3.

Dynamic ('stages of …') change theories (Prochaska/Diclemente, Rogers, Grol)

You may be familiar with the concept of 'stages of change' if you are a clinician who has ever tried to persuade a patient to give up smoking. Prochaska and Diclemente's original 'transtheoretical model' suggested that people move through a series of stages in seeking to change their behaviour: pre-contemplation, contemplation, preparation, action and maintenance [21]. In the first of these, the person is not even thinking about changing their behaviour. In the last, they have changed – but could slip back into their old habits.

The interventions needed to support behaviour change at each stage are different, so (according to this theory) the first step in influencing the individual is to establish their stage of change. It is also assumed that a person at the preparation stage will be more likely to change their behaviour than one at the pre-contemplation stage.

Everett Rogers, writing some decades earlier and addressing the adoption of innovations, produced a very similar stage-based model of change [22]. He proposed five stages: knowledge (in which the person becomes aware of the innovation), persuasion (in which they are actively seeking further information), decision (in which they decide whether to adopt the new behaviour), implementation (in which they begin to exhibit the new behaviour) and confirmation (in which they consolidate their decision, incorporating feedback on consequences and the reaction of peers).

Hall and Hord's concerns-based adoption model [23] is based on Rogers' stage-based model of innovation adoption. They proposed that the concerns of potential adopters change as they move from knowledge to implementation to confirmation. Specifically, before making the adoption decision, the main concerns are questions like, 'What is this innovation?', 'Will it help me?' and 'How much will it cost me?'; once the decision to adopt has been made, the main question is, 'How do I use this innovation?'; and during established use, it becomes, 'How can I modify this to make it more fit for purpose?'.

Richard Grol's team observed that whilst these stage models are conceptually appealing, there is, in reality, limited empirical support for either the transtheoretical model or the stages of change model depicted by Rogers in his diffusion of innovations theory. Incorporating ideas from these and similar staged approaches, Grol's team came up with a revised stages-of-change theory specifically designed to address guideline adoption by clinicians [24]. It consists of five stages:

1. **Orientation:** In which the potential adopter becomes aware of, and interested in, the new approach.
2. **Insight:** In which they come to understand the innovation and to understand the limitations of their current practice.
3. **Acceptance:** In which they develop a positive attitude to change, as well as the intention to change.
4. **Change:** In which they start exhibiting the new behaviour and confirm its value.
5. **Maintenance:** In which they work to embed the new practice into personal and organisational routines.

In Section 3.4, I will describe how Grol et al. built on this model to develop a stage-based series of interventions to support guideline adherence.

In sum, dynamic theories of change look at human behaviour as something that develops over time – and which may require continuing effort to become routinised and avoid slipping back into a previous pattern.

3.3 'Why don't clinicians follow guidelines?'

The (woefully incomplete) list of theories described briefly in Section 3.3 offers multiple ways of considering the age-old question of why clinicians do or don't follow evidence-based guidelines (or, perhaps more accurately, guidelines that someone believes to be evidence-based). But clinical behaviour is complex; it is situated in an organisational and professional context. For this reason, many scholars have sought to embed particular psychological theories in composite and/or multilevel frameworks that also address contextual issues.

In this section, I describe three overarching frameworks designed to explain clinician behaviour in relation to guideline adoption, developed by teams led by Susan Michie in the United Kingdom, Michael Cabana in the United States and Richard Grol in the Netherlands. Each was developed independently, although there is much overlap between them. None should be thought of as the definitive version of the truth.

Michie et al.'s taxonomy of behaviour change theories

Susan Michie was an early critic of empirical studies of guideline implementation, which she (rightly, in my opinion) viewed as based on a crude and undertheorised view of human behaviour. She led an expert group of health psychologists and health services researchers who produced, by consensus, a preliminary taxonomy of the key psychological domains and constructs needed for the implementation of evidence-based practice [25].

The twelve domains identified by this group were: (i) knowledge, (ii) skills, (iii) social or professional role and identity, (iv) beliefs about capabilities (embracing self-efficacy, but perhaps including other related constructs too), (v) beliefs about consequences, (vi) motivation and goals, (vii) memory, attention and decision processes, (viii) environmental context and resources, (ix) social influences, (x) emotion regulation, (xi) behavioural regulation and (xii) the nature of the behaviour. Each domain includes one or more theories of human behaviour.

Appendix B lists the many constructs (i.e. parts of theories) that were listed under these twelve headings in Michie et al.'s 2005 paper [25]. As you will see if you scan that list, the number of theories that are potentially relevant to the uptake and use of evidence by individuals is vast. Whilst all the constructs listed have merits, this early list is what I would call a brainstorm rather than a unifying theoretical perspective on how the different influences fit together. And it's too long for anyone to remember, which is why I have relegated it to an appendix!

Michie's team subsequently developed and extended their original list. Notably, they produced a 'behaviour change wheel' in which an inner wheel containing *theories of individual behaviour* was conceptualised as nested within a middle wheel of *interventions aimed at changing behaviour* (such as education, modelling, feedback, incentivisation and so on) and an outer wheel of *policies to support behaviour change* (including legislation, clinical guidelines, regulation and so on) [26]. Whilst I am ambivalent about the 'wheel' analogy, because it seems to imply a level of neatness that I've never encountered in the real world, I find the three conceptual levels (the individual, the intervention, the wider context) very useful.

In the behaviour change wheel, individual behaviour is depicted as dependent on three key factors: capability (what a person is capable of), motivation (the extent to which they want to behave in a particular way) and opportunity (the sum of enablers and constraints in the external world). This taxonomy of influences informed the diagram of why clinicians do not follow guidelines in Figure 3.2.

More recently, Michie's group has published a book listing 83 behaviour change theories relevant to health behaviour in patients or guideline adherence in clinicians [28]. It has even invited suggestions for theories it's missed – see its website, www.behaviourchangetheories.com.

Whilst I admire the work of Michie's group, I am a little concerned that the detailed theoretical analysis of human behaviour (using the constructs and theories listed in Appendix B) rarely happens in practice. Too often, students who find Appendix B too detailed reduce their analysis of complex behaviours in context to the capability/motivation/opportunity triad shown in Figure 3.2 – which in my view can be a dangerously oversimplified distillation of what is important. I do not think Michie and her group intended this to be the case, but I have seen a lot of naïve essays and academic papers that have misapplied this triad.

Cabana et al.'s model of barriers to physician adherence to guidelines

The first comprehensive review of why clinicians do not follow guidelines, by Michael Cabana's team in the United States, was published in 1996 and covered 76 primary studies [27]. The reviewers found some common factors across almost all studies: lack of awareness of the guideline, lack of familiarity with it, disagreement with the guideline's recommendations, a belief that one would be unable to follow the guideline (in Bandura's terms, 'low self-efficacy'), lack of motivation, low expectancy of positive outcomes and perceived external barriers beyond one's control. In Cabana et al.'s review, the most powerful influences were lack of awareness, low motivation and perceived external barriers.

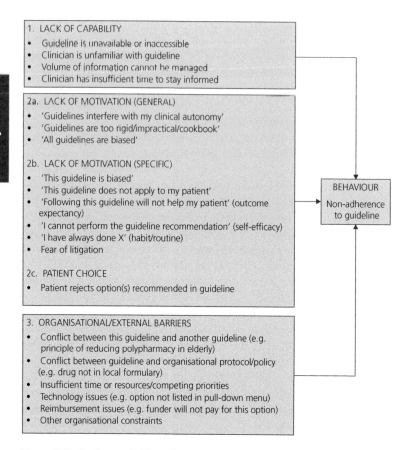

Figure 3.2 Barriers to clinician adherence to practice guidelines. *Source:* Adapted from Michie et al. [26] and Cabana et al. [27].

Figure 3.2 draws together Michie's widely-used Capability–Motivation–Opportunity–Behaviour (COM-B) framework [26] and Cabana's early framework of barriers to guideline adherence by clinicians [27]. Whilst the list of influences in Figure 3.2 is (I hope) a useful starting point to get you thinking about a particular scenario of non-adherence to guidelines, it is not intended as a comprehensive summary of all the evidence on this topic.

One problem with literature reviews is they can only give you the findings from what has been studied. It is clear from Cabana's review that certain factors are important, but all 76 primary studies that fed into the model in Figure 3.2 were designed very similarly: they started with the assumption that explanations would relate to the perceptions, awarenesses and capacities of the individual clinicians (including, in almost all of them, self-efficacy) – and that is what they found. Whilst these findings are not 'false', it is striking that there was no hint of the importance of such things as social networks and professional mindlines (see Section 10.3) – because early research had not yet identified these complex group-level phenomena as worthy of study.

It is also noteworthy that whilst Cabana and his team did an excellent job of identifying a list of *factors* (i.e. potential influencers) relevant to guideline adherence, they did not set out to develop *theory* (i.e. coherent explanations about how all the factors fitted together). Thus, this early work was a great start, but much remained to be done before clinician behaviour was adequately explained.

Grol's three-level model for guideline adherence
If Michie's team deserves the credit for producing a 'dictionary' of behaviour change theories, Richard Grol and his team from the Netherlands might be thought of as offering an accessible, unifying model of guideline adherence that can fit on a single page. Organising their constructs in a way that resonates with Michie's behaviour change wheel, they considered the influences on clinician behaviour at three levels:

1. **The individual professional:** Cognitive, educational, attitudinal and motivational (which I cover in the next section).
2. **The social context:** Including influences of peers on learning (next section), plus the wider social influences of professional and social networks, patient expectations and leadership (which I cover in Chapter 4).
3. **The organisational and economic context:** Here they included organisational innovativeness, approach to quality management, complexity, organisational learning and the wider economic context.

Table 3.2 summarises Grol's overarching model. Whilst I like this model overall, I prefer my own team's diffusion of innovations framework (see Chapter 5) for looking at the organisational and wider context.

In the next section, I consider some interventions for changing clinician behaviour that are (to a greater or lesser extent) supported by empirical evidence.

3.4 Interventions aimed at changing clinician behaviour

Interventions that prompt, reward, or feed back on behaviour
A high proportion of experimental studies of interventions to improve guideline adherence are based (or appear to be based) on the stimulus–response model that I criticised in Section 3.1. That is not to say the models

Table 3.2 Grol et al.'s summary of theories and models relating to implementing change in order to improve quality of care.

Theories/models	Important factors	Implications for implementation
Relating to individual professionals		
Cognitive	Mechanisms of thinking and deciding; balancing benefits and risks	Provide convincing evidence on the effectiveness and harms of interventions
Educational	Individual learning needs and styles	Involve professionals in improving current practice; define personal improvement plan
Attitudinal	Attitudes, perceived behavioural control, self-efficacy, social norms	Convince professionals of importance; show that they can do it and that others will follow
Motivational	Different motivational stages with different factors/barriers	Tailor interventions to different target groups (doctors, nurses, patients) within each field of care
Relating to social context		
Social learning	Incentives, feedback, reinforcement, observed behaviour of role models	Model best practice; give feedback on progress
Social network and influence	Existing values and culture of network, opinion of key people	Use opinion leaders in network to improve routines
Patient influence	Perceived patient expectations and behaviour	Involve patients actively in improving their care; promote and support self-management
Leadership	Leadership style, type of power, commitment of leader	Obtain commitment of management to making care more evidence-based
Relating to organisational and economic context		
Innovativeness of organisation	Extent of specialisation, decentralisation, professionalisation, functional differentiation	Take into account type of organisation; encourage teams to develop their own plans for change
Quality management	Culture, leadership, organisation of processes, customer focus	Reorganise processes for care; develop systems for continuous improvement
Complexity	Interactions between parts of a complex system, behavioural patterns	Focus on system as a whole; find main 'attractors' for improving care
Organisational learning	Capacity and arrangements for continuous learning in organisation	Encourage continuous exchange of expertise at all levels of the organisation
Economic	Reimbursement arrangements, rewards, incentives	Reward achievement of management targets

Source: Grol & Wensing [24]. Reproduced with permission of *The Medical Journal of Australia.*

are necessarily wrong, or that the interventions based on them are necessarily ineffective. But in my own view, the interventions tested were somewhat un-nuanced, and insufficient qualitative work was done to elucidate how they worked or why they failed to work. (Here's my bias: I was trained as a sociologist as well as a medical doctor, so I tend to value theory and I prefer real-world practice to be researched using detailed naturalistic designs.) That said, mainstream implementation science sets much store by these approaches, and most books on implementation of evidence start by reviewing them. So here goes.

The Cochrane Effective Practice and Organisation of Care (EPOC) group has supported a number of systematic reviews of randomised controlled trials of *reminders and prompts*. The overall conclusion from numerous studies is that reminders, whether delivered on paper or via computerised point-of-care prompts, are generally effective at improving adherence to guidelines in clinicians, although effects tend to be 'small to modest' [29,30].

The same is true of the much-cited systematic review of randomised trials of *audit and feedback*. This EPOC review included 140 trials of 'audit and feedback on' versus 'audit and feedback off', and again showed, overall, a 'small to modest' effect on professional practice in line with the guidelines [31].

I have to say I am cynical about these findings. The denominator population is not clinicians as a whole but clinicians who have agreed to be randomised in a study of adherence to a particular guideline – and who therefore probably have a positive attitude to the guideline. I also suspect that studies that demonstrated no effect (or a negative effect) may have been less likely to make it to publication.

It is not that I think reminders, prompts or feedback on performance are a bad idea. Quite the contrary. But my hypothesis is that if these interventions were optimised and carefully tailored to context, their effect would be moderate to large, not small to moderate!

Another intervention that might be viewed as behaviourist is the provision of *incentives or rewards* to clinicians who adhere to an evidence-based guideline or protocol. Once again, there is a systematic review by the Cochrane EPOC group showing that in randomised trials, the effect of financial incentives on physician performance ranged from zero to 'modest', and in each case, the reviewers commented that the methodological quality of many primary studies was poor [32–34].

Perhaps surprisingly, the use of financial incentives in this context is controversial. On the one hand, some studies have shown that paying clinicians to manage patients in a certain way (or penalising them for not doing so) improves adherence to the guidance in question. On the other hand, such policies have been dismissed as crudely behaviourist and even unethical

(Surely professionals should be treating patients according to best evidence, whether paid or not? Isn't it like paying children to do their homework rather than working to instil a genuine love of learning?). Studies suggesting that so-called 'pay-for-performance' schemes improve outcomes have been criticised for being too focused on short-term measurable benefits and failing to measure the unintended harms.

The classic example of this is the natural experiment of the Quality and Outcomes Framework (QOF) for UK general practice. Introduced in 2004, the QOF made a significant proportion of general practitioners' pay contingent on the achievement of certain targets derived from evidence-based guidelines. Some targets were linked to the process of care (e.g. recalling all their patients with known high blood pressure for an annual check-up) and some were linked to outcomes (e.g. ensuring that the blood pressure of these patients was below a certain level).

Early research on the impact of the QOF appeared to demonstrate that it not only improved both the process and outcome of care in the designated disease areas, but also reduced inequalities because its effects were largest on people from the most deprived backgrounds (the health-conscious middle-classes being, perhaps, the low-hanging fruit) [35]. But subsequent studies, summarised in a systematic review by Steve Gillam and colleagues, suggested two critical qualifiers to this finding [36]. First, improvements in QOF-designated disease areas were achieved at the expense of deterioration in diseases that were *not* included in the QOF. Second, the more doctors focused on achieving their 'QOF targets', the less time or attention they gave to their patients' presenting complaints – in other words, care shifted from being patient-centred to being clinician-centred, and even QOF-centred.

In sum, paying clinicians to provide evidence-based care in one area of practice is no guarantee of improving care overall. In some cases, it produces benefits in one (monitored) part of the system at the expense of causing harms in another part of the system. To those who view incentives as the golden route to improving practice, don't forget the unintended (and usually unmeasured) consequences.

Interventions that seek to improve knowledge

It is self-evident that if a clinician does not know about a guideline or recommendation, he or she cannot change practice in line with it. But clinicians are not empty buckets, and providing them with information may or may not mean that it gets read, understood, assimilated and used to change practice. Common sense suggests that sending written information to clinicians will work in some situations some of the time, and the research base is almost meaningless unless we know quite a bit about the clinical and wider context for a knowledge-based intervention. But as you have already seen from the previous subsection, the implementation science literature is dominated by randomised trials of intervention on versus intervention off, with absent or limited qualitative components, and the primary studies on such experiments have been grouped together in broad-brush EPOC reviews.

Here are the key findings from some of those reviews:

- Trials of *printed education materials* suggest that they have a small to modest effect on clinical practice some of the time, but the qualitative data in included studies were so weak that 'we could not comment on which [printed educational material] characteristic influenced their effectiveness' [37].
- Trials of *educational meetings* for clinicians suggest that, compared to no meetings, they have a small positive effect on professional practice, which may be translated to improved patient outcomes, but that such meetings are generally ineffective at inducing 'complex behaviours' [38].

In sum, knowledge-focused and instructional interventions improve practice, but – on average – not by much. Such approaches are not going to change the world.

Given the apparent importance of negative attitudes towards guidelines in studies of barriers to adherence with them, there is surely much potential in interventions aimed at changing attitudes. Such interventions rely heavily on social influence and are discussed further later in this section.

Interventions that promote the use of heuristics

Given the significant evidence base on the superiority of System-1 (analogical) over System-2 (deductive) reasoning (Section 3.2), it is surprising that, at the time of writing, there is not a single review on the Cochrane Database that mentions the word 'heuristics' in the title, abstract or keywords!

Arguably, this is an example of anchoring bias (Table 3.1). The EBM movement set out to rationalise clinical practice, and purists in the movement might classify the use of heuristics as 'second best solutions' [39]. Yet the emerging empirical evidence base appears to show that in general, when we use heuristics, decisions are both more accurate and more timely. Marewski and Gigerenzer, for example, offer a simple heuristic (Figure 3.3) for deciding whether to admit a patient to a coronary care or standard bed that ignores most of the information in the full evidence-based Bayesian decision tree – but which performs at least as well as the latter in assigning patients to the most appropriate bed [40]. I rarely use the phrase 'more research is needed', but my own view is that the development, introduction and evaluation of heuristic reasoning tools should be a high priority for the next era of EBHC.

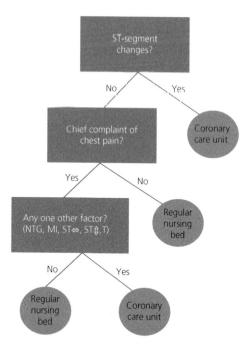

Figure 3.3 'Fast-and-frugal' heuristic for deciding whether a patient should go to the coronary care unit or a standard nursing bed. If there is a certain anomaly in the electrocardiogram (the so-called ST segment), the patient is immediately sent to the coronary care unit. Otherwise, a second predictor is considered, namely whether the patient's chief complaint is chest pain. If it is not, a third question is asked. This question is a composite one: whether any of five other predictors is present. *Source:* http://www.dialogues-cns.org/publication/heuristic-decision-making-in-medicine/, accessed October 2016. Adapted from Gigerenzer, G. (2007). *Gut Feelings: The Intelligence of the Unconscious.* New York, NY: Viking Press; 2007, and Green, L., & Mehr, D.R. (1997). What alters physicians' decisions to admit to the coronary care unit? *Journal of Family Practice,* **45,** 219–226.

Interventions that promote adult (on-the-job) learning

Some years ago, Michael Green published a paper on graduate training for evidence-based practice which concluded that such training needed to occur 'where the rubber meets the road' – that is, in the clinic and at the bedside – since the adult learning cycle (Figure 3.1) implies the need for some, if not all adults to learn through practical experience and problem-solving, as well as through abstract reasoning [41].

I was surprised, then, when researching this chapter, not to find more empirical studies of on-the-job training in the skills of evidence-based practice. Medical and nursing students typically learn their critical appraisal skills in the classroom, in a way that is strongly oriented to passing assessments.

The standard format for teaching the same skills to graduates is the journal club – in which one member typically presents a paper, perhaps relating to a patient seen recently. A recent systematic review suggested that journal clubs improve the ability to appraise journal articles but that their effect on patient care is entirely unknown [42].

In short (and unless I've missed the literature entirely), the application of the principles of adult learning to the design of interventions to improve professional practice in line with best evidence is currently – somewhat ironically – an evidence-free zone.

Interventions that promote social influence

The EPOC group has undertaken a number of reviews of studies that compared some form of social influence against a control intervention. The most important of these are:

- Trials of *educational outreach* ('academic detailing'), in which clinicians were visited in their workplace by an independent adviser (typically an academic) to discuss an aspect of practice [43]. Broadly, these studies demonstrated a statistically significant change in practice, especially in relation to prescribing (although rather less in other kinds of clinical behaviour), when compared either with no intervention or with audit and feedback. The absolute change in practice achieved from these visits tended to be modest, and few studies looked at the medium- or long-term sustainability of the change.
- Trials of *local opinion leaders*, in which practitioners were randomised to receive a visit from a respected local colleague in the same specialty or either no intervention or a different intervention (usually audit and feedback) [44]. Overall, such trials demonstrated a modest but statistically significant change in behaviour in the direction of the evidence-based standard, although the primary studies were very heterogeneous (i.e. they studied different things in different ways) and in one or two cases the influence of the 'opinion leader' appeared to be negative rather than positive.

My own view is that social influence is not best studied using experimental designs, and we need more naturalistic (qualitative) studies of who really influences whom in the real world. I expand on this theme in Section 10.2 when I talk about social network analysis.

Sequential interventions tailored to the intended adopter's stage of change

If we base an intervention on dynamic change theories, it makes sense to use a sequential approach. Table 3.3 shows the 10-step approach that Grol et al. [24,45] developed based on the five stages of change in clinician behaviour described in Section 3.2 (orientation, insight, acceptance, change and maintenance).

As Table 3.3 shows, Grol et al. [24,45] recommend a series of interventions, initially aimed at creating awareness of the existence of a new guideline or approach to practice, then (once awareness is achieved) shifting to encouraging clinicians to reflect on their own practice and gain insight into the gap between that and the evidence-based recommendation. Once this is achieved, the intervention should move to helping the practitioner develop a positive attitude to change and an intention to change (including self-efficacy in the ability to change). Once practitioners have motivation and confidence, interventions should focus on supporting them to make small-scale changes in their practice and observe the results. Finally, there is the important step of supporting the maintenance and routinisation of the new practice in the organisation.

Grol et al.'s [24,45] sequential model has intuitive appeal, and many of the theories of human behaviour reviewed in this section can be identified in it. However, this model has (to my knowledge) not been prospectively tested as a complex intervention in practice.

In conclusion, human behaviour is a complex phenomenon, not least because it is embedded in a social context. In the last 10 years in particular, much progress has been made in identifying, classifying and combining psychological theories to produce a model of how clinicians behave in relation to evidence-based guidance. But the current evidence base remains incomplete, and we are still some way short of a multilevel theoretical framework that will allow us to make sense of the multiple dimensions of why clinicians do the things they do (and resist doing other things). I should also declare an interest: my own team is working on an alternative multilevel framework, which I hope to include in a second edition of this book!

3.5 Ten tips for influencing how people behave

1. Don't think of people as empty buckets or blank slates
I started this chapter with a quote on how human actors actively engage with potential innovations (either positively or negatively). Far too much research on behaviour change ignores the diverse, complex and creative ways in which humans engage with new ideas, practices or technologies. Strategies to influence humans must, first and foremost, acknowledge this aspect of humanness.

Table 3.3 Grol et al.'s sequential approach to implementation based on a stages-of-change theory of clinician behaviour.

Proposed intervention	Potential barriers to change	Potential ways to overcome barriers
Orientation stage		
Promote awareness	Unfamiliar, does not read literature, no contact with colleagues	Distribute brief messages via all types of channel; approach key figures and networks
Stimulate interest	No sense of urgency, does not see it as relevant	Attention-catching literature or website; personal approach and explanation; confrontation regarding performance
Insight stage		
Create understanding	No knowledge; information too complex and/or too extensive	High-quality instruction materials, concise messages; information based on problems in practice; regular repetition of message
Develop insight into own routines	Limited insight; overestimation of own performance	Simple methods of audit and feedback on performance; comparison of data with peers
Acceptance stage		
Develop positive attitude to change	Sees disadvantages, has doubts about value or developers, not attracted to change	Adapt innovation to wishes of target group, with local discussion and consensus; discuss resistance; provide good scientific arguments; involve key individuals and opinion leaders
Create positive intentions/ decision to change	Has doubts about feasibility success, and own efficacy	Have peers demonstrate feasibility; detect bottlenecks, seek solutions and propose feasible objectives for change
Change stage		
Try out change in practice	Not starting, no time, lack of skills, does not fit into fixed routines	Extra resources, support, training in skills, redevelopment of care processes, temporary support or consultants, information materials for patients
Confirm value of change	Insufficient success, negative reactions of others	Devise plan that includes feasible objectives for change, inventory of bottlenecks and the seeking of solutions
Maintenance stage		
Integrate new practice into personal routines	Relapse, forgetting	Monitoring, feedback and reminder systems; integration in routine care plans and local protocols
Embed new practice in organisation	No support, no budget	Provide resources, support from top management, organisational measures, rewards, payment for specific tasks

Source: Grol & Wensing [24] and Grol et al. [45]. Originally from Grol, R., & Wensing, M. (2005). Characteristics of successful innovations. In: *Improving Patient Care; The Implementation of Change in Clinical Practice* (eds R. Grol, M. Wensing & M. Eccles). Oxford, Elsevier, pp. 60–70.

2. Think fast – and slow

Section 3.2 introduced the work of Daniel Kahnemann, who reminded us that most of our thinking consists of heuristics and pattern recognition. If you base your efforts to influence clinicians on the assumption that they will assimilate all the information provided and make rational decisions derived from that information, you have not understood a very basic principle of human thinking. We need fewer inch-thick guidelines and more fast-and-frugal heuristics.

3. Know your cognitive biases

It is a delicious irony that there are way too many cognitive biases to commit to memory. But that does not mean we can ignore these biases. You should know the basics – Box 3.1 reminds you that the main biases can be grouped under four overarching headings: too much information, not enough meaning, the need to act fast and the challenge of what to remember.

4. Challenge stock theories of behaviour change

In Section 3.2, I made the provocative suggestion that people who research clinician behaviour and how to change it are sometimes guilty of following fads. How many authors based their study on the theory of planned behaviour because that was what the last study used? How many used a self-efficacy scale without engaging with the wider theoretical basis of self-efficacy as described by Bandura? Don't be a lemming. Think carefully about your theoretical perspective – and choose an appropriate approach, even if it is different from the ones other people have used.

5. Get familiar with the basics of learning theory

If you plan to run any kind of educational course or training programme, take a look at Bloom's learning domains and Kolb and Knowles' adult learning theory in Section 3.2. The more you get your head around these approaches, the less likely you are to commit the three most common sins in adult education: (i) limiting your programme to 'talk and chalk'; (ii) overloading your learners with unnecessary detail; and (iii) assessing exclusively through recall.

6. Think of behaviour change as occurring in stages …

Section 3.2 introduced various stages of change models – including Prochaska and DiClemente's transtheoretical model and Rogers' stages of innovation adoption. It makes sense to tailor what you do to influence behaviour to which stage the intended adopter is in. Table 3.3 shows how a time dimension allows you to sort out the various theories and models and select the most appropriate for a given individual's stage of adoption.

7. … and also as influenced at different levels

As well as giving your analysis a time dimension, give it some texture. Look at Grol et al.'s simple three-tier model of influences (individual, social, organisation) on guideline adherence in Section 3.3 and how different theories map to different levels (Table 3.2). I hope you will be inspired to move beyond static, one-dimensional accounts of behaviour ('the rat went down the left hand side of the maze') to produce richer pictures in three dimensions.

8. Distinguish 'factors' (barriers, facilitators) from explanations

In Section 3.3 I introduced several useful models for considering why clinicians do not follow guidelines. But I also warned that such models were not really theories as such – they were frameworks for remembering a host of different potential influences operating at different levels. To explain why a particular clinician (or group of clinicians) is not following a particular guideline in a particular context, we also need a unifying theory of how the different factors influence one another and evolve over time. In my own view, we need fewer 'factor analysis' studies (which produce a numerical estimation of the contribution of each factor to a predefined outcome) and more *narrative explanations* that make sense of what is happening.

9. Understand the limitations of experimental trials of interventions to change behaviour

In Section 3.4, I listed the main findings from several Cochrane reviews of randomised trials of different interventions aimed at increasing guideline adherence by clinicians (reminders, prompts, audit and feedback, incentives/rewards, printed educational materials, educational meetings, educational outreach and local opinion leaders). All were found to help – although the impact of each was modest. But as I explained in that section, I am concerned that the study design of controlled experiment stripped out the contextual influences that were key to the outcome. I referred forward to later sections in this book, where I consider studies of what actually happens in real-world settings.

10. Build capacity

Most researchers have spent years learning the basic principles of good research in their discipline, acquiring the skills of searching and critical appraisal and developing the ability to distil the key findings from a lengthy research report. They then expect non-researchers to access, understand and use research publications with no training or support.

A fundamental principle of research uptake and use in any organisation is to *develop staff*. This is not just about providing general training in research-related skills for staff at almost all levels; it is also about endorsement of the value of research knowledge for the organisation's mission (e.g. from the chief executive, senior management and clinical directors) and development of the *organisation's* capacity to identify, take up and circulate relevant new knowledge – a complex phenomenon known as *absorptive capacity*. I discuss all these concepts in more detail in Chapter 5.

References

1. Greenhalgh, T., Robert, G., Macfarlane, F., Bate, P., & Kyriakidou, O. (2004). Diffusion of innovations in service organizations: systematic review and recommendations. *The Milbank Quarterly*, **82**(4), 581–629.
2. Skinner, B. (1974). *About Behaviorism*. New York, Vintage.
3. Kahneman, D. (2011). *Thinking, Fast and Slow*. New York, Macmillan.
4. Gigerenzer, G. (2014). *Risk Savvy: How to Make Good Decisions*. New York, Penguin.
5. Gigerenzer, G., & Brighton, H. (2009). Homo heuristicus: why biased minds make better inferences. *Topics in Cognitive Science*, **1**(1), 107–143.
6. Gigerenzer, G., & Selten, R. (2002). *Bounded Rationality: The Adaptive Toolbox*. Cambridge, MA, MIT Press.
7. Gigerenzer, G., & Gaissmaier, W. (2011). Heuristic decision making. *Annual Review of Psychology*, **62**, 451–482.
8. Blumenthal-Barby, J.S., & Krieger, H. (2015). Cognitive biases and heuristics in medical decision making: a critical review using a systematic search strategy. *Medical Decision Making*, **35**(4), 539–557.
9. Greenhalgh, T., Kostopoulou, O., & Harries, C. (2004). Making decisions about benefits and harms of medicines. *BMJ*, **329**(7456), 47–50.
10. Ajzen, I. (1991). The theory of planned behavior. *Organizational Behavior and Human Decision Processes*, **50**(2), 179–211.
11. Fishbein, M., & Ajzen, I. (1975). *Belief, Attitude, Intention and Behavior: An Introduction to Theory and Research*. Reading, MA, Addison-Wesley.
12. Kortteisto, T., Kaila, M., Komulainen, J., Mäntyranta, T., & Rissanen, P. (2010). Healthcare professionals' intentions to use clinical guidelines: a survey using the theory of planned behaviour. *Implementation Science*, **5**, 51.
13. McEachan, R.R.C., Conner, M., Taylor, N.J., & Lawton, R.J. (2011). Prospective prediction of health-related behaviours with the Theory of Planned Behaviour: a meta-analysis. *Health Psychology Review*, **5**(2), 97–144.
14. Godin, G., Bélanger-Gravel, A., Eccles, M., & Grimshaw, J. (2008). Healthcare professionals' intentions and behaviours: a systematic review of studies based on social cognitive theories. *Implementation Science*, **3**(36), 1–12.
15. Sniehotta, F.F., Presseau, J., & Araújo-Soares, V. (2014). Time to retire the theory of planned behaviour. *Health Psychology Review*, **8**(1), 1–7.
16. Bloom, B.S. (1956). *Taxonomy of Educational Objectives: The Classification of Education Goals by a Committee of College and University Examiners*. London, Longmans.
17. Kolb, D.A. (1984). *Experiential Learning: Experience as the Source of Learning and Development*. Englewood Cliffs, NJ, Prentice-Hall.
18. Elwyn, G., Greenhalgh, T., & Macfarlane, F. (2000). *Groups: A Hands-On Guide to Small Group Work in Education, Management and Research*. Oxford, Radcliffe.

19. Bandura, A. (1976). *Social Learning Theory*. Englewood Cliffs, NJ, Prentice-Hall.

20. Sherer, M., Maddux, J.E., Mercandante, B., Prentice-Dunn, S., Jacobs, B., & Rogers, R.W. (1982). The self-efficacy scale: construction and validation. *Psychological Reports*, **51**(2), 663–671.

21. Prochaska, J.O., & DiClemente, C.C. (1992). Stages of change in the modification of problem behaviors. *Progress in Behavior Modification*, **28**, 183.

22. Rogers, E.M. (2010). *Diffusion of Innovations*, 5th edn. London, Simon and Schuster.

23. Hall, G., & Hord, E. (1974). The Concerns-Based Adoption Model: A Developmental Conceptualization of the Adoption Process Within Educational Institutions. Austin, TX, University of Texas.

24. Grol, R., & Wensing, M. (2004). What drives change? Barriers to and incentives for achieving evidence-based practice. *Medical Journal of Australia*, **180**(6 Suppl.), S57.

25. Michie, S., Johnston, M., Abraham, C., Lawton, R., Parker, D., & Walker, A. (2005). Making psychological theory useful for implementing evidence based practice: a consensus approach. *Quality and Safety in Health Care*, **14**(1), 26–33.

26. Michie, S., van Stralen, M.M., & West, R. (2011). The behaviour change wheel: a new method for characterising and designing behaviour change interventions. *Implementation Science*, **6**(1), 42.

27. Cabana, M.D., Rand, C.S., Powe, N.R., Wu, A.W., Wilson, M.H., Abboud, P.-A.C., & Rubin, H.R. (1999). Why don't physicians follow clinical practice guidelines?: a framework for improvement. *JAMA*, **282**(15), 1458–1465.

28. Michie, S., West, R., Campbell, R., Brown, J., & Gainforth, H. (2014). *ABC of Behaviour Change Theories: An Essential Resource for Researchers, Policy Makers and Practitioners*. London, Silverback Publishing.

29. Arditi, C., Rège-Walther, M., Wyatt, J.C., Durieux, P., & Burnand, B. (2012). Computer-generated reminders delivered on paper to healthcare professionals; effects on professional practice and health care outcomes. *Cochrane Database of Systematic Reviews*, **12**:CD001175.

30. Shojania, K.G., Jennings, A., Mayhew, A., Ramsay, C.R., Eccles, M.P., & Grimshaw, J. (2009). The effects of on-screen, point of care computer reminders on processes and outcomes of care. *Cochrane Database of Systematic Reviews*, **3**:CD001096.

31. Ivers, N., Jamtvedt, G., Flottorp, S., Young, J.M., Odgaard-Jensen, J., French, S.D., et al. (2012). Audit and feedback: effects on professional practice and healthcare outcomes. *Cochrane Database of Systematic Reviews*, **6**:CD000259.

32. Scott, A., Sivey, P., Ait Ouakrim, D., Willenberg, L., Naccarella, L., Furler, J., & Young, D. (2011). The effect of financial incentives on the quality of health care provided by primary care physicians. *Cochrane Database of Systematic Reviews*, **9**(9):CD008451.

33. Flodgren, G., Eccles, M.P., Shepperd, S., Scott, A., Parmelli, E., & Beyer, F.R. (2011). An overview of reviews evaluating the effectiveness of financial incentives in changing healthcare professional behaviours and patient outcomes. *Cochrane Database of Systematic Reviews*, **7**(7):CD009255.

34. Rashidian, A., Omidvari, A.H., Vali, Y., Sturm, H., & Oxman, A.D. (2015). Pharmaceutical policies: effects of financial incentives for prescribers. *Cochrane Database of Systematic Reviews* (8):CD006731.

35. Doran, T., Fullwood, C., Kontopantelis, E., & Reeves, D. (2008). Effect of financial incentives on inequalities in the delivery of primary clinical care in England: analysis of clinical activity indicators for the quality and outcomes framework. *The Lancet*, 372(9640), 728–736.

36. Gillam, S.J., Siriwardena, A.N., & Steel, N. (2012). Pay-for-performance in the United Kingdom: impact of the Quality and Outcomes Framework – a systematic review. *The Annals of Family Medicine*, 10(5), 461–468.

37. Giguère, A., Légaré, F., Grimshaw, J., Turcotte, S., Fiander, M., Grudniewicz, A., et al. Printed educational materials: effects on professional practice and healthcare outcomes. *Cochrane Database of Systematic Reviews*, 10:CD004398.

38. Forsetlund, L., Bjorndal, A., Rashidian, A., Jamtvedt, G., O'Brien, M.A., Wolf, F., et al. (2009). Continuing education meetings and workshops: effects on professional practice and health care outcomes. *Cochrane Database of Systematic Reviews*, 2:CD003030.

39. Bodemer, N., Hanoch, Y., & Katsikopoulos, K.V. (2015). Heuristics: foundations for a novel approach to medical decision making. *Internal and Emergency Medicine*, 10(2), 195–203.

40. Marewski, J.N., & Gigerenzer, G. (2012). Heuristic decision making in medicine. *Dialogues in Clinical Neuroscience*, 14(1), 77–89.

41. Green, M.L. (2000). Evidence-based medicine training in graduate medical education: past, present and future. *Journal of Evaluation in Clinical Practice*, 6(2), 121–138.

42. Ahmadi, N., McKenzie, M.E., MacLean, A., Brown, C.J., Mastracci, T., & McLeod, R.S.; Evidence-Based Reviews in Surgery Steering Group (2012). Teaching evidence based medicine to surgery residents – is journal club the best format? A systematic review of the literature. *Journal of Surgical Education 2012*, 69(1), 91–100.

43. O'Brien, M.A., Rogers, S., Jamtvedt, G., Oxman, A.D., Odgaard-Jensen, J., Kristoffersen, D.T., et al. (2007). Educational outreach visits: effects on professional practice and health care outcomes. *Cochrane Database of Systematic Reviews*, 4:CD000409.

44. Flodgren, G., Parmelli, E., Doumit, G., Gattellari, M., O'Brien, M.A., Grimshaw, J., & Eccles, M.P. (2011). Local opinion leaders: effects on professional practice and health care outcomes. *Cochrane Database of Systematic Reviews*, 8:CD000125.

45. Grol, R.P., Bosch, M.C., Hulscher, M.E., Eccles, M.P., & Wensing, M. (2007). Planning and studying improvement in patient care: the use of theoretical perspectives. *The Milbank Quarterly*, 85(1), 93–138.

Chapter 4 **Groups and teams**

4.1 Introduction: no man (or woman) is an island

Before you read any further, make a list of the different groups you belong to. Here's a selection of mine: doctors (my profession); Oxford academics (my main job); multidisciplinary primary health care teams (my other job); carers of elderly relative (a family role); long-distance walking club (a hobby); charity trustees (a committee role); cancer survivors (a patient role). In these groups, I enact many different identities and behave in different ways – because the groups have different purposes and different unwritten rules ('norms') for how their members are expected to behave.

What is a group? I particularly like John Hunt's definition:

> *A group is any number of people who are able to interact with each other, are psychologically aware of each other, and who perceive and are perceived as being members of a team.* [1]

The terms 'group' and 'team' are not quite interchangeable, but I will treat them as such for the purposes of this chapter.

Using this definition, the groups/teams we need to consider in relation to implementing evidence-based healthcare (EBHC) include (but are not limited to):

- the handful of people with whom we work most closely to deliver care (e.g. what used to be called the 'firm' in a hospital and is now sometimes referred to as a 'clinical microsystem');
- people we work with as part of the formal structures and governance of an organisation (e.g. committee, governing body, board of examiners);
- people working on a one-off project with us (e.g. sometimes known as a 'task and finish' group), which may include people outside our organisation;

How to Implement Evidence-Based Healthcare, First Edition. Trisha Greenhalgh.
© 2018 John Wiley & Sons Ltd. Published 2018 by John Wiley & Sons Ltd.

- colleagues within our organisation with whom we share a wider interest (e.g. members of a journal club);
- people within our profession who support us and who we support (as I describe in Section 10.3, support groups – of midwives, physiotherapists, general practitioners and so on – increasingly exist online);
- people beyond our workplace and across professions with whom we share a topic interest (e.g. diabetes, evidence-based medicine);
- support and lobbying groups of patients and carers (see Sections 6.3 and 10.4).

Very little healthcare these days is delivered by a single individual working in isolation. Most of us know and use the acronym MDT ('multidisciplinary team'). Each of us – including the patient and carer – contributes something towards the overall care package. Everyone on the team has to know at least something about what the others are doing, respect that contribution and adapt their own input accordingly. Evidence to support effective multidisciplinary care cannot just sit in one individual's head. It has to be shared, collectivised, negotiated and put into practice by the team as a whole.

Like any other group, an MDT is not merely a collection of individuals. It has a purpose, a set of norms (expectations for acceptable and unacceptable behaviour), some rules of engagement and a division of roles. The people in the team support and motivate one another; they draw out one another's strengths and compensate for one another's weaknesses. Those teams that operate effectively (see Box 4.1) can achieve more than the sum total of their individual members' contributions.

The size of a working group is key to its success. Too small, and you will have too few members to achieve the skill mix required for an interdisciplinary task. Too large, and it gets messy. Some years ago, John Øvretveit demonstrated, in the context of delivering community-based healthcare, that it is increasingly difficult to achieve co-ordination and co-operation between members as the size of a group increases [2].

The number of possible interactions between a group's members is determined by the mathematical formula $I = n\,(n-1)/2$, where I = number of interactions and n = number of members. In a group of three people, for example, there are three possible interactions: A-B, A-C and B-C. With four people, the number of possible interactions increases to six: A-B, A-C, A-D, B-C, B-D and C-D. But with 10 members, there are 45 potential interactions (which is one reason why, in a large group, everyone needs to direct their questions and comments through the chair). Most of us have been in the situation of feeling stressed and confused simply because the group we are trying to work in is too large.

> **Box 4.1 Characteristics of effective groups**
>
> **The members**
> - work co-operatively, not competitively;
> - 'get along' with one another;
> - take incentives and rewards collectively, not individually;
> - are aware of the nature of the group process and the stages of group development.
>
> **The group**
> - is not too large (ideally five or six members);
> - has autonomy to address its task(s);
> - has an appropriate mix of knowledge and skills;
> - has an effective leader or facilitator;
> - is adequately resourced in terms of time and administrative support.
>
> **The task**
> - involves all members, draws on the skills of different individuals and requires co-ordination;
> - is concrete, rather than abstract;
> - has a precise statement of objectives, a definitive beginning and end, and measurable indicators of success.
>
> **The context**
> - the group operates within a wider context of a supportive organisation or community;
> - the physical and material environment is adequate (e.g. space, quiet);
> - the expectations placed on the group are appropriate and achievable.
>
> *Source: Adapted from Hunt [1].*

Traditionally, groups are said to go through a series of phases: forming (getting together), storming (a phase of conflict during which the rules are disputed), norming (agreeing the rules by which the group will operate) and conforming (following those rules and doing the work of the group). Where the group is an established and formal part of an organisation (as in the primary healthcare team), group norms may have been set years ago and – whilst they will continue to evolve and be challenged – the main phase of the group is now 'conforming'. Indeed, the roles and routines of a long-established group are an important source of organisational stability (but see the section on 'Routinisation and Sustainability' in Section 5.6).

Strong groups and teams have a clearly recognisable identity that transcends the identities of the individual members (think of the All Blacks rugby team or a world-leading neurosurgery team). In a sense, such groups have 'personalities' that are not merely the sum (or the average) or the person-alities of their members. The rest of this chapter considers how leaders and facilitators might harness the combined skills, values and ethoses of a group or team to optimise its work, and in particular how to lead or facilitate the group process in the implementation of best evidence. I end the chapter with a sum-mary of tips for constructing, leading and facilitating groups and teams.

4.2 Leadership

In my personal view, the literature on leadership has an exceptionally high noise to signal ratio – in other words, there's a lot of poor research and even more unsubstantiated speculation on the topic. This section draws on many sources, including a book called *Groups* that I co-authored, in which the leadership chapter was written mainly by Glyn Elwyn [3].

What is a leader? Here is a personal (subjective) definition. For me, a leader is someone I can look up to; someone I am prepared to follow (hence, some-one whose judgement I trust) and someone who has integrity (hence, someone who will attend to the moral dimension of our work). He or she should have relevant experience and expertise (but not necessarily be *the* expert on a topic). He or she should be intelligent, quick-thinking, hard-working and positive. I want them to be able to articulate a vision on behalf of our team – and to talk about that vision in a way that inspires me. If my leader wants me to commit to something, I want them to show their own commitment first.

I also want my leader to understand their team members as individuals, support them and encourage them. The leader should have excellent 'chair-person' skills – for example, clarifying a task, setting a democratic ethos for contributions, and keeping all members to task and time. They will need high emotional intelligence, so that they can assess how their followers are reacting to a situation. I want my leader to generate and sustain team spirit and ensure that team members (even the junior ones) feel they can speak up and raise concerns. In short, I want my leader to have excellent personal qualities *and* to attend skilfully and wisely to the task, the individuals and the team as a whole.

This list of characteristics, which is entirely subjective and the result of a personal brainstorm, aligns broadly with the evidence from organisational sociology on the process of leadership: leaders create *authority structures* to oversee and coordinate work (and, particularly, the processes of innovation and change); they create *psychological safety* ('a shared belief that interper-sonal risks will not be punished'); and they promote *team stability* (in short, if the team members are confident in their leader, they feel secure as a team and are less likely to leave and get a new job somewhere else) [4].

The conventional taxonomy of leadership divides leaders into charismatic, inspirational and transformational [3]. *Charismatic leaders* use their powerful personalities and charm to gather followers. They are dominant, self-confident individuals who hold strong conviction for their beliefs and engender high levels of loyalty, identification and trust. *Inspirational leaders* motivate people to commit to a cause, set high standards and goals for themselves, work hard and strive to do a better job. They typically lead by example, working hard and setting high standards for themselves. *Transformational leaders* act more like facilitators, taking a democratic approach and motivating people to develop themselves and rise above their individual aims to think more widely about the needs of the group or organisation. Other authors have added a fourth category to this taxonomy: *laissez-faire leaders*, who (arguably) do not really lead at all. They wish to allow the group to set its own agenda, and hence give little direction on either task or team processes.

Many years ago, Kurt Lewin undertook an experiment on schoolboys, in which he identified three boys with different leadership styles (democratic, autocratic and laissez-faire) and invited them to lead groups in a construction task [5]. The groups with a democratic leader (who encouraged participatory decision-making) and an autocratic leader (who made all major decisions themselves) produced comparable products, but the latter group enjoyed the task much less and eventually became resentful and unmotivated. The group with the laissez-faire leader was neither productive nor happy. This widely cited experiment is food for thought: it suggests that strong leadership is better than weak leadership, but it also raises more questions than it answers about the fitness for purpose of different leadership styles in different contexts.

Paul Gorman adapted the generic taxonomy of leadership styles to the specific context of healthcare improvement teams, and came up with the following variants [6]:

- **The superhero leader:** Aloof, thinking big thoughts but with an eye on the distant horizon. Tends to be surrounded by a 'personality cult' to which his (usual) success is attributed. Tends to have an autocratic, directive style.
- **The democratic leader:** Focused on people and staff, with a consensual and discursive management style. Does not seek personal gain but serves as a voice for the wider team and a catalyst for group action.
- **The bureaucratic leader:** An expert in the organisational machine, focused on structures and systems. Has a leadership style characterised by pragmatism and attention to detail.
- **The reluctant leader:** Achieves a leadership role by default rather than design, and given the choice would not be there at all. Once in the post, may mature into one of the other leadership styles (most usually, democratic). Includes many clinical directors (doctors who take on a temporary or permanent management role in a hospital).

Chapter 4

Gorman's taxonomy raises (but does not directly address) the question of gender in leadership. Are superhero and bureaucratic leaders more likely to be men? Are democratic and reluctant leaders more likely to be women? And does it matter? In the light of the huge push in UK healthcare to develop more women as leaders (both because it's fair and because they are seen as offering a new *style* of leadership) [7], I have summarised the evidence on gender in Box 4.2. But before we get too tied up on that topic, evidence suggests that (i) gendered leadership styles are more evident in laboratory experiments than in the real world; and (ii) the most successful leaders of either gender tend to possess features of both 'male' and 'female' leadership styles and to adapt their style flexibly to suit the situation. It is, of course, the style of leadership and its appropriateness to context that matters, not the presence or absence of a Y-chromosome.

Gender aside, contemporary healthcare organisations (and, incidentally, many other organisations in the modern world) are almost invariably complex, fast-changing and unpredictable. It has been argued (although by no means proven beyond doubt) that men and women who exhibit a classically 'female' leadership style will have an advantage – and confer that advantage on to their teams [12].

Gender (and gendered leadership styles) were hot topics in the leadership literature a few years ago, but they have to some extent been superseded by research on the importance of *distributed leadership* in healthcare organisations and systems. Some years ago, I worked with Allan Best on a systematic review of large-system change in healthcare organisations [13]. One key finding was that because health systems are so complex and because change often needs to occur across departments, organisations and even sectors, a single person cannot, individually, shoulder the entire burden of leadership. Rather, leadership must be negotiated and shared amongst several people – and, indeed, almost everyone needs to lead something. I return to the notion of distributed leadership in Section 11.1, where I talk about complexity and leadership. For an authoritative review of distributed leadership, see Richard Bolden's paper, 'Distributed Leadership in Organizations: A Review of Theory and Research' [14].

It has also been argued that distributed leadership, along with characteristics I have associated with a 'female' leadership style, is needed to support compassionate care in healthcare organisations [15]. Paquita de Zulueta reasons as follows:

> *Strategies for developing compassionate health care leadership in the complex, fast-moving world of today will require a paradigm shift from the prevalent dehumanizing model of the organization as*

Box 4.2 Gender and leadership style

Whilst leaders of either gender may exhibit any trait or style, evidence suggests that, in general, male leaders are more likely to be:

- confident;
- authoritative;
- decisive;
- firm;
- formal;
- unemotional;
- task-oriented.

In contrast, research studies in the commercial sector have found that, compared to men, women leaders:

- tend to be people-oriented rather than task-oriented;
- command less;
- interact, consult and include more;
- share their uncertainties more;
- share more power and seek win–win;
- draw productively on their own emotions and those of their staff;
- move more easily and flexibly between formal and informal spaces.

These different styles are not inherently good or bad. A 'male' leadership style tends to be most appropriate when there is/are:

- a stable organisational structure;
- well-defined hierarchies and roles;
- clear tasks and boundaries; and
- a stable external environment.

In contrast, a 'female' leadership style is generally more appropriate when there is/are:

- a changing organisational structure;
- a changing external environment;
- poorly defined hierarchies and roles;
- changing tasks with fuzzy boundaries;
- a high level of uncertainty and low level of agreement on what the task is.

Source: Based on research by (mostly) American business and management academics [8–11].

---

machine to one of the organizations as a living complex adaptive system. It will also require the abandonment of individualistic, heroic models of leadership to one of shared, distributive, and adaptive leadership. 'Command and control' leadership, accompanied by stifling regulation, rigid prescriptions, coercive punishments, and/or extrinsic rewards, infuses fear into the system with consequent disempowerment and disunity within the workforce, and the attrition of innovation and compassion. It must be eschewed. Instead, leadership should be developed throughout the organization with collective holistic learning strategies combined with high levels of staff support and engagement. [15]

There are remarkably few empirical research studies of what makes good leadership in a clinical context. One that I rather like is a small focus-group study of what constitutes excellence from anaesthetists in relation to patient safety [16]. The focus groups were made up of anaesthetic nurses, who described features of excellence. It was clear that excellence was not merely the technical skill of inducing (and reversing) anaesthesia. In addition, the lead anaesthetist displayed (to a greater or lesser extent) the following leadership characteristics:

- a structured, responsible and focused way of approaching work tasks;
- a clear and informative style, briefing the team about the action plan before induction;
- a humble attitude to the complexity of anaesthesia, admitting his or her own fallibility where appropriate;
- patient-centredness, making personal contact with the patient before the induction;
- fluency in the practical procedures of anaesthesia without losing overview; and
- calmness and clarity in critical situations, being able to change to a more directive leadership style when circumstances required it.

These findings illustrate a number of themes covered earlier in this section. Leadership is a complex and elusive phenomenon. As the authors of the Swedish study point out, these aspects of the anaesthetist's work often attract little attention in specialist training, yet they are as crucial to patient safety as technical skills. The authors suggest that 'role models' should be studied more carefully with a view to promoting better leadership in the profession. This is an excellent idea: instead of studying leadership (in the abstract), we should study *leaders* (real people, leading real teams) and learn from their approach. Howard Gardner did this in an excellent (and very readable) book, covering leaders from Margaret Mead to Robert Oppenheimer [17].

4.3 Facilitation and team learning

Facilitating (which means 'helping' or 'enabling') is not the same as leading. Leaders have followers; facilitators have teams with whom they are working – and sometimes, teams who have hired them to help address a particular project or challenge. In relation to the work of groups and teams, the term 'facilitation' refers to both support for learning (both individual learning and team learning) and support for action (e.g. helping people mobilise the resources they need to achieve a goal). In particular, good facilitation supports the effective linking of learning and action.

One of the most popular models of evidence implementation in teams is the PARIHS (Promoting Action on Research Implementation in Health Services) framework, developed by a team consisting mostly of academic nurses, including Alison Kitson, Gill Harvey and Jo Rycroft-Malone [18,19]. PARIHS proposes a three-way interaction between evidence, context and facilitation. Depending on the strength of evidence and features of context, the type of facilitation needed differs. I discuss PARIHS in more detail in Appendix A, where I cover frameworks more generally.

To unpack the notion of facilitation, I went exploring and discovered an excellent article in *Implementation Science* by Whitney Berta and team entitled 'Why (We Think) Facilitation Works' [20].

To explain Berta et al.'s theory of facilitation, I first need to digress into organisational learning theory (originally proposed by Argyris and Schön [21]). Most of what I have to say about organisations is in Chapter 5, but so-called 'organisational' learning theory belongs in this chapter because the social process of learning occurs largely in a team (or what Berta et al. call 'microsystem') setting. People in organisations appear to learn – or not – in small groups and teams of colleagues with whom they work closely.

Organisational learning theory conceptualises organisations, and the microsystems within those organisations, as having a (greater or lesser) capacity to learn. Facilitation is viewed as operating via its impact on this team-level learning. Argyris and Schön proposed that people have mental maps (also known as 'scripts', 'schemas' or 'tacit structures') that guide them on how to act in particular situations, informing how they plan, implement and review their actions. It is these mental maps that guide people's actions, rather than the theories of change they explicitly espouse. Few people are aware of the schemas they use until these are revealed through the facilitation process.

Argyris and Schön proposed two contrasting theories to explain the link between how we think and how we act. *Theories in use* are the mental maps or schemas just described. *Espoused theories [of action]* are the words we use to convey to others what we do and why we do it. Espoused theories and theories in use are often incongruent (in other words, what drives our action is not what we think is driving our action). Furthermore, if the consequences of our action align with what we expected to happen, this tends to affirm (perhaps subconsciously) our theory-in-use. If they do not, we become confused and seek an explanation.

Organisational learning (or – my preferred term – team learning) occurs when we reflect on the difference between what we planned and expected to happen in a particular situation and what actually happened. Typically, people then come up with a different approach that helps to achieve the team's original goal. This is what Argyris and Schön call *single-loop learning*. As a team undertakes this essential process of reflection on action, it may also identify things that might be corrected at a system level – so-called *double-loop learning* ('when error is detected and corrected in ways that involve the modification of an organization's underlying norms, policies and objectives' [21]). It might also learn something about the process of team learning itself (*triple-loop learning*), but let's put that third level aside for now.

Berta et al. consider that facilitation is the process by which single-, double- and triple-loop learning are supported in organisations through reflection on action. It is worth quoting directly from their paper:

> *Organizational learning is a social process. Members of an organization interact to construct meaning and knowledge about action-outcome relationships and about effects of the organization's context (learning environment) on those relationships. Some learning manifests as observable changes in worker behaviours and work routines. Other learning is not observable, such as learning that leads to decisions not to change. Individuals in organizations learn in a social context of other learners, with prior learning and accrued knowledge embedded in that context. Organizational learning therefore is more than the sum of what individuals know and learn, and it can persist well beyond the tenure of individuals. Learning that persists may be captured in explicit and encoded formal policies and procedures, in information and data collection systems, or in less explicit forms likened to reservoirs in an organization's memory, informal communication channels, culture, and behavioural norms.*

According to these authors, facilitation is a proactive, social process oriented to achieving evidence-informed practice change. It incorporates dimensions of project management, leadership, relationship building and communication. It has three main components: (i) the facilitator role (and activities linked to this); (ii) the process of facilitation; and (iii) the outcomes of facilitation (which may include double- and triple-loop learning, as well as the directly intended change).

Facilitation involves working with teams to help them reflect on practices, and thereby understand gaps in performance and identify where changes can be made. This may include incongruent mental maps, attitudes and assumptions, ways of working or deficiencies in (team) knowledge or skills. The facilitator helps identify how to address these barriers, improve communication channels and monitor progress. An important component of the facilitation process is working on team relationships and promoting trust, including creating the psychological safety to allow members (even junior ones) to raise concerns and thereby surface questions about the gap between theories-in-action and espoused theories.

In sum, facilitation is a widely used approach to supporting the implementation of evidence-based practice in teams and organisations. The process of facilitation is based on a theory of team learning and collective action. This in turn rests on the notion of shared schemas for action and the dissonance between what team members think they are doing (and achieving) and what they are actually doing and achieving. Importantly, team learning includes learning about the issue at hand (single-loop), learning about how to correct and improve things in the system more widely (double-loop) and learning about team learning itself (triple-loop).

4.4 Empirical studies of leadership and facilitation

This section considers some studies of leadership and facilitation in the implementation of evidence. As always, different research methods will address different kinds of question. Experimental studies (such as randomised trials) can be designed to ask, 'If we add leadership component X, will it change outcome Y?', although staff may experience such experiments as contrived. Naturalistic studies (such as ethnography of real-world healthcare teams) can ask, 'What is really going on in terms of leadership in this team?' In this section, I describe an example of a randomised trial that was billed as having tested leadership as a variable in an evidence implementation study [22] and a qualitative case study of what kind of leadership and facilitation actually worked in evidence implementation across a sample of hospitals [4].

A randomised controlled trial by Anita Huis and colleagues (including the internationally rated implementation science expert Richard Grol) addressed the question, 'Can we improve nurses' compliance with hand-hygiene guidance using a targeted leadership and social influence intervention?' [22]. These authors randomised 67 hospital wards to intervention or control arms. All wards were offered a 'state-of-the-art' package comprising things that would tend to promote implementation of the hand-washing guidance: (i) excellent facilities to support regular hand-washing; (ii) education on the

Chapter 4

benefits of regular hand-washing; (iii) reminders; and (iv) feedback on performance. The first of these is a prerequisite, of course; the last three, as summarised in numerous Cochrane reviews (see Section 3.4), are all evidence-based ways of improving performance in line with the evidence.

In addition to this, wards in the intervention arm also received 'a team and leaders-directed strategy ... aimed at addressing barriers at team level by focussing on social influence in groups and strengthening leadership'. This intervention, consisting of three 90-minutes facilitated sessions to set goals, identify barriers and review feedback data, was based on social influence theory, social learning theory and something the authors called 'leadership theory' (the first two are covered in Section 3.2, whilst leadership was covered in Section 4.2, although I dispute that there is a single 'leadership theory'). The study aimed to achieve (v) active commitment and initiative from ward managers; (vi) modelling by informal leaders on the ward; and (vii) the setting of norms and targets within the team.

After 6 months, compliance with hand-hygiene guidance had improved from 23 to 42% in the control group and from 20 to 53% in the intervention group; these changes were sustained 6 months later, and differences between groups were statistically significant.

The authors' conclusion was that effective leadership is an important component of implementation of evidence in healthcare teams and that it can be improved with strategies directed at the team leader. I do not disagree that that conclusion is compatible with the data, but I worry that the study's authors have reduced leadership (a complex, fuzzy and largely unmeasurable quality) to a variable and attempted to manipulate that variable experimentally. Were they really measuring leadership? Or was the 'thing' they were measuring a combination of additional facilitated education sessions plus some contrived role modelling? Whatever it was, it worked, so I take my hat off to this team. But as someone who tends to prefer naturalistic studies to experimental ones, I was unconvinced of the study's central claim to have *measured the impact of leadership*.

In a very different research genre, and with an explicit focus on the team learning process, organisational sociologist Amy Edmondson undertook a classic qualitative study of the introduction of minimally invasive cardiac surgery (MICS) in surgical units in 16 different hospitals across the United States [4]. Published in 2001, this study looked at a procedure that is now commonplace but which at the time was highly innovative and fitted poorly with existing team routines. The researchers conducted ethnographic observation of team meetings and operations, and interviews with all involved staff over the study period. There was huge variation in the uptake of MICS across the sample of 16 units 6 months later. The researchers classified units into 'successful' ($n = 7$) and 'unsuccessful' ($n = 7$); two units were intermediate and excluded from the final analysis.

Edmondson et al.'s evidence on 'success' and 'failure' in implementing MICS is summarised in Figures 4.1 and 4.2, respectively. They found that the introduction of a complex team innovation required four steps:

1. enrolment (selecting which members of the team should be involved);
2. training (learning, as a team, to deliver the innovation);
3. trial (doing it for real);
4. reflection (considering what had gone well and troubleshooting things that had not).

In teams that successfully introduced MICS, enrolment was characterised by a number of active leadership and facilitation strategies used to select members, set a frame for team learning and justify the rationale, as well as by corresponding active buy-in from members (something we might call effective followership), as illustrated in the first panel in Figure 4.1.

In contrast, leaders of unsuccessful teams approached the enrolment phase very differently (Figure 4.2): they did not select team members strategically, placed less emphasis on team learning and framed the task as a need to learn, *as individuals*, to use a plug-in technology. In subsequent phases, leaders of successful teams showed up for training, continued to emphasise the *team* learning element (and especially reflection on action), created psychological safety and encouraged people to participate and raise concerns. Leaders of unsuccessful teams were unengaged themselves and did little to motivate or support participation by their staff. Ironically, but perhaps unsurprisingly, leaders whose priority was writing an academic paper about the innovation tended to fail to implement it!

Edmondson et al.'s study supports an important conclusion: leaders who command respect from their team members and who put effort into supporting the people, the task and the team – that is, those who actively *lead* and *facilitate* their teams – are far more likely to succeed in transforming services than those whose actions are best described using a different verb ('selecting', 'allocating', 'commanding', 'testing'). In my view, Edmondson's study also illustrates that it is *good leaders* – that is, real people with integrity, courage, emotional intelligence and so on – and not the abstracted variable of *leadership* that gets results from teams (see my note about Howard Gardner's book in the previous section).

Innovation was successfully adopted when ....

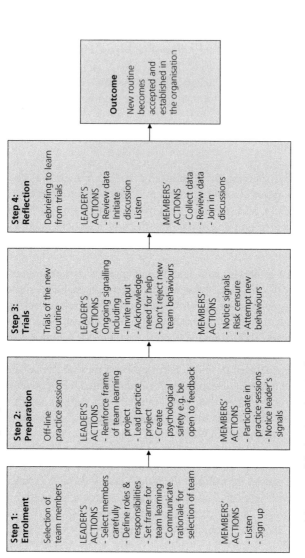

Figure 4.1 Features of the successful adoption of minimally invasive cardiac surgery (MICS). *Source:* Edmondson et al. [4]. Reproduced with permission of SAGE Publications.

Innovation was not successfully adopted when ....

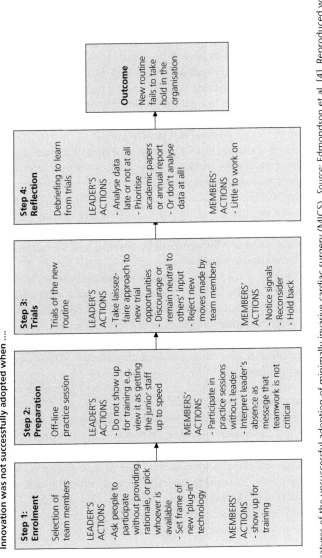

Figure 4.2 Features of the unsuccessful adoption of minimally invasive cardiac surgery (MICS). *Source*: Edmondson et al. [4]. Reproduced with permission of SAGE Publications.

4.5 Ten tips for leading and facilitating teams

As always, there is no magic formula, but there are some useful rules of thumb.

1. Understand the mathematics of group work

See what I said in Section 4.1 on the difficulties of achieving effective group or teamwork if a group is too large. If your 'team' is 20 or 30 people, you will almost certainly need to generate subgroups with particular tasks or remits, although this does not preclude you all meeting together for some things (e.g. informal social events or a periodic review meeting).

2. Attend to the team's physical and material needs

As John Hunt reminded us (Box 4.1), any group with work to do needs space, time, resources and regular breaks. Groups that lack the time to prepare or reflect, or those who are asked to do their business in a space that is cramped or not private, will function poorly even when well facilitated (but especially when that is not the case).

3. Assess the context in which you will be working, and the implications for the preferred leadership style

Look back at Section 4.2. Is your team and the setting in which it operates stable, predictable and well-defined? Are tasks and roles clear and unchanging? If so, a directive and task-oriented leadership style may be appropriate. Or is your team and/or the wider organisation in a state of flux, with an unstable external environment and unclear task(s), and with the only certainty being changeability? If so, a more democratic and people-oriented leadership style is likely to work better.

4. Don't be a wuss

We can argue all day about which leadership style is best for which setting (please do – you can start with what I said in Section 4.2 and add more evidence of your own). But I suspect you would agree that the literature is consistent on one thing: some leadership is better than no leadership. If you are in charge of something, get a grip. You need to select your team, articulate the task, support individual and group learning and drive through the change process. You may lean naturally to a more autocratic (hierarchical, directive) or democratic (participatory) style, but don't behave as if you're in a commune.

5. Select your team carefully, and justify to everyone why people have been included

Most tasks in healthcare organisations need a mix of team members. If you are setting up a new task group, it may or may not be appropriate to use a formal appointment process and advertise the different roles using a job description and person specification. Whether people are appointed formally or informally, Edmondson et al.'s study (Section 4.4) clearly shows that those who know they have been selected for a particular skill or quality tend to engage better with the group process than those who are unsure why they have been picked.

6. Clarify the task objectives and measures of success with your team

This is basic project management (see John Hunt's advice again, Box 4.1). With your team, make progress from a vague statement of a distant goal ('to introduce evidence-based guidelines') to objectives that are SMART (specific, measurable, achievable, results-focused and time-bound) – such as 'to ensure that all patients seen in hospital A with condition X are managed according to guideline Y by time Z'. The tools and techniques in Appendix A, such as process mapping and driver diagrams, may be helpful.

7. When facilitating a team, take account of task(s), context and team preparedness

This maxim is based on the PARIHS framework, introduced briefly in Section 4.3 and explained in more detail in Appendix A. In relation to the specific task and objective, what aspects of context are relevant? Is the organisation or department likely to embrace change in this area – and if not, what might stand in the way? Is the evidence (research, local audits, the patient experience) consistent and uncontested? Are individuals aware of the evidence, accepting of its key messages and committed to change? If not, what are their main learning needs and how might these be addressed? In sum, where does the team/organisation lie on the PARIHS diagnostic grid (Figure A.7) – and what are the implications for facilitation?

8. Attend to people issues as well as task issues

This is another key dimension of both leadership (Section 4.2) and facilitation (Section 4.3). Are all team members clear about their roles and confident in their ability to fulfil them? Do they understand what is expected of them? Do they like and trust one another? If not, what are their misgivings and what can you do to address them? Have the team members had enough time to get to know one another? Do the more junior members, in particular, experience psychological safety (e.g. would they speak out if they had concerns)? Are you, the leader, setting an excellent example in terms of your own attendance, commitment and contribution?

9. Give plenty of feedback (both 'hard' and 'soft')

As noted in Chapter 3, feedback on performance is one of the best-evidenced strategies by which to improve uptake and use of evidence. Evaluating progress is partly about defining and using agreed metrics of success (it is the third step in the simple definition of strategy: (i) Where are we going?; (ii) How are we going to get there?; (iii) How are we going to know we've got there?). Feedback is also about providing the qualitative human feedback and support required to maintain team spirit and ensure that individuals feel valued. Putting effort into something with no feedback on how you're doing is demotivating and stressful. Conversely, praise and thanks, given both collectively and individually, build commitment. If you're shy about this, practice saying, out loud, phrases like 'You're doing a great job, folks' or 'I'd particularly like to thank Ramesh for the graphs he drew, which I'm going to use in my report to the board'.

10. Attend to the cycle of team learning (single-, double- and triple-loop)

As noted in Section 4.3, identifying a gap between what you should be doing and what you are doing (single-loop learning) is often fairly straightforward. Making a change to improve an outcome may also be relatively easy. But can you get your team to rise above the immediate goal to think about the underlying *system* issues (double-loop learning)? And at the same time, can you encourage them to think about the process of team learning so that they come to value it, contribute to it and seek to improve it (triple-loop learning)?

References

1. Hunt, J. (1993). Groups in organizations. In: *Managing People at Work*. New York, McGraw Hill.
2. Øvretveit, J., & Borsay, A. (1994). Coordinating community care: multidisciplinary teams and care management. *Ageing and Society*, **14**(1), 141.
3. Elwyn, G., Greenhalgh, T., & Macfarlane, F. (2000). *Groups – A Hands-On Guide to Small Group Work in Education, Management and Research*. Oxford, Radcliffe.
4. Edmondson, A.C., Bohmer, R.M., & Pisano, G.P. (2001). Disrupted routines: team learning and new technology implementation in hospitals. *Administrative Science Quarterly*, **46**(4), 685–716.
5. Lewin, K., Lippitt, R., & White, R.K. (1939). Patterns of aggressive behavior in experimentally created 'social climates'. *The Journal of Social Psychology*, **10**(2), 269–299.
6. Gorman, P. (1998). *Managing multi-disciplinary teams in the NHS*. London, McGraw-Hill Education.
7. Ovseiko, P.V., Edmunds, L.D., Pololi, L.H., Greenhalgh, T., Kiparoglou, V., Henderson, L.R., et al. (2016). Markers of achievement for assessing and monitoring gender equity in translational research organisations: a rationale and study protocol. *BMJ Open*, **6**(1), e009022.
8. Eagly, A.H., Johannesen-Schmidt, M.C., & Van Engen, M.L. (2003). Transformational, transactional, and laissez-faire leadership styles: a meta-analysis comparing women and men. *Psychological Bulletin*, **129**(4), 569.

9. Eagly, A.H., & Johnson, B.T. (1990). Gender and leadership style: a meta-analysis. *Psychological Bulletin*, **108**(2), 233.

10. Blanchard, K., & Miller, M. (2014). *The Secret: What Great Leaders Know and Do.* Oakland, CA, Berrett-Koehler Publishers.

11. Ibarra, H., Ely, R., & Kolb, D. (2013). Women rising: the unseen barriers. *Harvard Business Review*, **91**(9), 60–66.

12. Eagly, A.H. (2007). Female leadership advantage and disadvantage: resolving the contradictions. *Psychology of Women Quarterly*, **31**(1), 1–12.

13. Best, A., Greenhalgh, T., Lewis, S., Saul, J.E., Carroll, S., & Bitz, J. (2012). Large-system transformation in health care: a realist review. *The Milbank Quarterly*, **90**(3), 421–456.

14. Bolden, R. (2011). Distributed leadership in organizations: a review of theory and research. *International Journal of Management Reviews*, **13**(3), 251–269.

15. de Zulueta, P.C. (2016). Developing compassionate leadership in health care: an integrative review. *Journal of Healthcare Leadership*, **8**, 1–10.

16. Larsson, J., & Holmström, I.K. (2012). How excellent anaesthetists perform in the operating theatre: a qualitative study on non-technical skills. *British Journal of Anaesthesia*, **110**(1), 115–121.

17. Gardner, H.E. (1995). *Leading Minds: An Anatomy of Leadership*. New York, Basic Books.

18. Kitson, A., Harvey, G., & McCormack, B. (1998). Enabling the implementation of evidence based practice: a conceptual framework. *Quality in Health Care*, **7**(3), 149–158.

19. Kitson, A.L., Rycroft-Malone, J., Harvey, G., McCormack, B., Seers, K., & Titchen, A. (2008). Evaluating the successful implementation of evidence into practice using the PARiHS framework: theoretical and practical challenges. *Implementation Science*, **3**(1), 1.

20. Berta, W., Cranley, L., Dearing, J.W., Dogherty, E.J., Squires, J.E., & Estabrooks, C.A. (2015). Why (we think) facilitation works: insights from organizational learning theory. *Implementation Science*, **10**(1), 141.

21. Argyris, C., & Schön, D. (1978). *Organizational Learning: A Theory of Action Perspective*. Reading, MA, Addision-Wesley.

22. Huis, A., Schoonhoven, L., Grol, R., Donders, R., Hulscher, M., & van Achterberg, T. (2013). Impact of a team and leaders-directed strategy to improve nurses' adherence to hand hygiene guidelines: a cluster randomised trial. *International Journal of Nursing Studies*, **50**(4), 464–474.

Chapter 4

Chapter 5 **Organisations**

5.1 The diffusion of innovations model

Back in 2003, my team was contracted by the UK Department of Health to summarise the literature on how innovations spread from one healthcare organisation to another. The research was intended to solve what had been called the 'Six West problem' – that is, when the staff on ward Six West developed an innovation that was beneficial to patients, why was this innovation so slow to spread to ward Six East just across the corridor, let alone to other wards and other hospitals?

For the purposes of our review, we defined an innovation as follows:

An innovation in health service delivery and organisation is a set of behaviours, routines and ways of working, along with any associated administrative technologies and systems, which are:
a. perceived as new by a proportion of key stakeholders
b. linked to the provision or support of health care
c. discontinuous with previous practice
d. directed at improving health outcomes, administrative efficiency, cost-effectiveness, or the user experience
e. implemented by means of planned and co-ordinated action by individuals, teams or organisations.
Such innovations may or may not be associated with a new health technology.

This definition embraces (but is not limited to) new drugs and devices (which often need a change in clinic or theatre routines to support them); new research findings with implications for the way services are organised; educational, lifestyle or other complex interventions; guidelines, protocols and care pathways; and new staff roles (such as the introduction of physician assistants or nurse prescribers).

How to Implement Evidence-Based Healthcare, First Edition. Trisha Greenhalgh.
© 2018 John Wiley & Sons Ltd. Published 2018 by John Wiley & Sons Ltd.

We found that the empirical research relevant to our research question was messy, incomplete, inconsistently reported and dispersed across a lot of different disciplines. Indeed, we had to develop a new methodology for systematic review, called meta-narrative review, to unpick all the different research traditions that had addressed aspects of the Six West problem, often using different methodologies and generating findings that were not entirely consistent with one another. We published the main findings in 2004 [1] and the original methodology of meta-narrative review in 2005 [2]. The full, detailed review came out as a book in 2005 [3]. More recently, an international Delphi panel developed quality standards and publication guidance for meta-narrative review as part of the RAMESES (Realist and Meta-narrative Evidence Synthesis – Evolving Standards) programme [4].

Our 2004 review of the diffusion of innovations (which quickly became the most highly cited paper I've ever written) did not turn up any quick fixes, and neither did the update we produced in 2010 [5]. But we did produce a multilevel model for thinking about how service-level innovations emerge; how they spread – and why they often fail to spread – as ideas and practices between individuals and organisations; and how (if at all) organisations assimilate and routinise them. The model – which, although not perfect, has stood the test of time and been applied to hundreds of different organisational innovations in healthcare over the years – is shown in Figure 5.1. It has nine components, which I will outline briefly in this section before going on to discuss the organisational elements in more detail.

The first component is the innovation itself, which is more likely to be taken up if its attributes in the eyes of potential adopters included such things as relative advantage, low complexity, compatibility with values and ways of working, trialability, observability, potential for reinvention and (for technologies) ease of use. I discussed these attributes in Section 2.4.

The second component is the potential adopters of the innovation – what I called 'people' in Chapter 3. As noted in that chapter, our model considered the adoption of evidence by people as an active and complex process involving learning and persuasion. Different people have different personalities, are more or less technologically minded, are more or less risk-averse and have different past experiences.

The third component is social influence, which is key to individual adoption decisions. Social influence includes the role of opinion leaders (high-status peers or experts whom we seek to copy), champions (people who back a product and support its introduction) and boundary-spanners (people who bring ideas and examples from elsewhere), all of whom are discussed in more detail in Section 10.2. In our review, we found that much adoption occurs by *diffusion*, which is traditionally understood as an essentially passive process of copying others, although in reality it usually involves extended processes

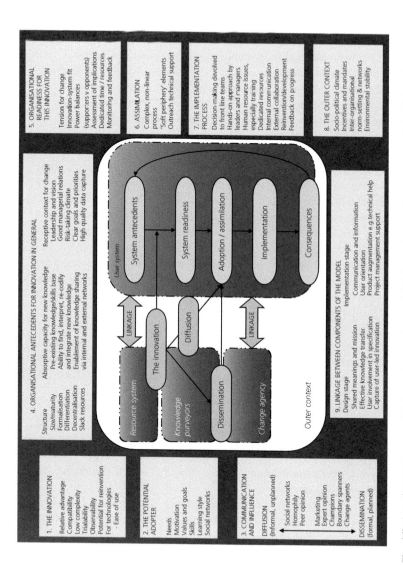

Figure 5.1 The diffusion of innovations model. *Source:* Greenhalgh et al. [1]. Reproduced with permission of John Wiley & Sons.

of social learning (see Chapter 3): experimentation, interaction with other users (or potential users), failure and reinvention (i.e. adapting the innovation to suit a local context). Our review also found that active dissemination strategies can be highly effective if opinion leaders and champions are played to their strengths.

The fourth, fifth, sixth and seventh components of the model relate to the organisation into which the innovation is taken up (or not), which is the main focus of this chapter. The fourth addresses general features of the organisation. Some organisations are inherently better set up to identify and assimilate innovations than others. Organisational innovativeness is partly determined by structural features (such as size and resources), which are covered in Section 5.2. But more importantly, organisations differ hugely in their overall propensity to take up new knowledge (their *absorptive capacity*) and in their *receptive context for change* (including things like organisational culture and climate). These important constructs are addressed in Section 5.3.

The fifth component is how the model stands in relation to a particular innovation. Even when an organisation supports service-level innovation in general, its readiness for any *particular* innovation depends on prevailing pressures for change: whether the supporters of the innovation outnumber its opponents and have the influence to drive it forward. This in turn depends on the supporters' capacity to articulate a credible positive narrative for the implications of the innovation for the organisation, and the degree of innovation–system fit (e.g. the extent to which the innovation aligns with the core business of the organisation). These considerations are discussed further in Section 5.4.

The sixth component of the model is the process of assimilation (the organisational-level parallel to individual adoption). The term 'adoption' is generally (but not universally) used to refer to uptake of an innovation by individuals, and 'assimilation' to uptake by an organisation. Service-level innovations can be thought of as having a 'hard core' (the essential features of the innovation) and a 'soft periphery' (aspects of the wider organisation which need to adapt to accommodate the innovation into business as usual). This is covered in more detail in Section 5.4.

The seventh component is implementation and routinisation within the organisation, which can be done well or badly – as described in Sections 5.5 and 5.6. Devolution of decision-making to front-line teams, hands-on input from leaders and senior managers, bespoke training (especially of teams in a real-world, on-the-job setting), targeted resources, effective channels (formal and informal) for internal communication and accurate and timely feedback on progress can all make or break an effort to introduce complex innovation even when there is broad-based support for it (and especially when there is not).

Chapter 5

The eighth component is the external ('outer') context for innovation. The wider environment (i.e. the prevailing economic and political context) and the behaviour of other organisations in the same sector (and the extent to which the index organisation is linked with, and influenced by, the same) can exert a powerful influence on the organisation-level adoption decision. The components of the model relating to inter-organisational networks and the wider sociopolitical context are discussed later in the book (see in particular Chapter 9 on policy and Chapter 10 on networks).

Finally, the ninth component is the dynamic relationship between the first eight; this is as critical to innovation success as any of the components individually. Linkage (communication, consultation, dialogue and so on) between different organisations and sectors does not lead automatically to consensus or a self-evident way forward, but it may lead to better orientation amongst stakeholders and to the development of a shared vocabulary with which to negotiate effectively. This important 'whole-system' consideration is the subject of Chapter 11.

5.2 Structural determinants of organisational innovativeness

Much of the early research on organisational assimilation of innovations took the form of a one-shot survey (typically sent to the chief executive, who passed it on to someone else) asking questions about an organisation's size, structure, financial status and so on. The responses from dozens or hundreds of organisations were fed into a computer, and statistical analysis was used to find which of the elements accounted for each organisation's 'innovativeness' – that is, whether or not it had adopted a particular innovation.

This research can be criticised for using a relatively weak methodology (retrospective one-off surveys don't sit very high in the hierarchy of evidence), but with that caveat in mind, the findings of such surveys are remarkably consistent. In a nutshell, an organisation will assimilate innovations more readily if:

- it is *large* (organisational size is almost certainly a proxy for other determinants, including slack resources and functional differentiation);
- it is *mature* (i.e. it has been around for some years and developed a niche in its core business);
- it is *functionally differentiated* (i.e. it is divided into semi-autonomous departments and units);
- it is *specialised* (some of the organisation and management literature uses the term 'complexity', which generally refers to a composite measure of the degree of specialisation, functional differentiation and professional knowledge);

- it has *decentralised* decision-making structures (i.e. its different component units can decide whether or not to adopt something new without asking for approval from a central board, committee or decision-maker);
- it has *slack resources* available to be channelled into new projects.

Healthcare organisations, certainly in secondary care, tend to be large, mature (in the sense meant here) and highly functionally differentiated (the X-ray department, for example, is quite separate from the cardiology department and the patient records department). The extent of decentralisation of decision-making varies a lot between organisations, even in the UK National Health Service (NHS) (which, contrary to popular belief, is not one organisation, but many, disparately connected organisations). As in all organisations, senior managers may be more or less likely to micromanage their heads of department and require all decisions to be passed up the line for approval. My advice: if you trust your staff, leave them alone to do their job (and if you don't trust them, what are they doing in charge of a department anyway?).

The extent of slack resources (i.e. a budget that can be rapidly and strategically deployed to fund the assessment and piloting of a new idea or product) is increasingly a rate-limiting factor in public-sector healthcare organisations. The continuing pressure on these organisations to make 'efficiency savings' means that budgets have been pared down to the bare minimum required to deliver the current service and there is precious little available to spend on new ideas. Importantly, even when an innovation itself is free (e.g. an idea for running a clinic differently), there will be significant costs associated with the work of assimilating and implementing it (see Sections 5.4 and 5.5). Many excellent ideas have hit the sand through a dearth of slack resources.

5.3 Absorptive capacity and receptive context

If you ask only about structural features, you will generate findings relating only to structural features. So whilst factors like size, differentiation and slack resources are important, they are often less important than the 'softer' (i.e. more human and more difficult to measure) dimensions of the organisation that were not, in general, included in early research on organisational innovativeness.

Perhaps the most important of those softer dimensions is absorptive capacity. This construct, originally developed by business and management academics [6], was a key component of our original diffusion of innovations model, but I have learnt a lot more about it in recent years from Cathy Howe and Gill Harvey, who have been studying absorptive capacity in hospitals. This section draws particularly on their work.

Chapter 5

Absorptive capacity seeks to explain how well or badly organisations are at learning, problem-solving and taking up innovations. It is defined as 'a set of organisational routines and processes by which [organisations] acquire, assimilate, transform and exploit knowledge to create a dynamic organisational capacity' [6]. It consists of four overlapping processes (Table 5.1 and Figure 5.2).

First, an innovative organisation must have the capability to *acquire* knowledge from outside its own walls. Knowledge acquisition happens when an organisation already has a stock of internal knowledge on relevant topic areas, when it has relevant infrastructure (e.g. high-quality systems for capturing and managing data) to allow it to bring in more knowledge and when it invests in measures to seek out and capture knowledge (e.g. by sending staff on courses, carrying out horizon-scanning work, implementing dedicated knowledge roles and so on). Of course, knowledge acquisition in a particular area will depend on the external antecedents of what knowledge is 'out there' and how easy it is to get hold of – a topic I cover in more detail in Chapter 10.

Second, the organisation members must be able to *assimilate* that knowledge. It's no good sending one member of staff on a course or asking them to search the Internet if they are incapable of achieving understanding of the topic they have been asked to research. Individuals must be carefully selected and supported to ensure active learning that leads to understanding.

Third, the organisation needs to *transform* the knowledge from the dry, abstract formats in which it is typically packaged to the practical, workable forms in which it can actually be applied. A crucial aspect of knowledge transformation is the extent to which staff in the organisation are supported to come together to hear about new ideas, discuss their interpretations and concerns ('What does this mean for me?') and reframe their mental models

Table 5.1 Absorptive capacity.

Step/dimension	Components	Contribution
Knowledge acquisition	Prior investments	Scope of search
	Prior knowledge	Perceptual schemas
	Intensity	New connections
	Speed	Speed of learning
	Direction	Quality of learning
Knowledge assimilation	Understanding	Interpretation
		Comprehension
		Learning
Knowledge transformation	Internalisation	Synergy
	Conversion	Reframing
		Bisociation
Knowledge exploitation	Use	Core competencies
	Implementation	Harvesting resources

Source: Adapted from Zahra & George [6].

Absorptive capacity (AC) framework (adapted from Lane et al. 125).

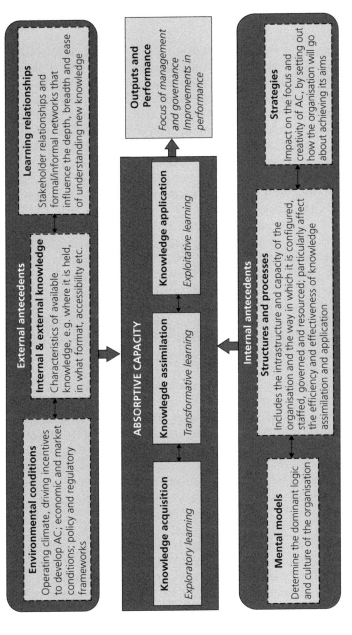

Figure 5.2 A model of absorptive capacity in healthcare. *Source:* Harvey et al. [7], adapted from Lane et al. [8]. Reproduced with permission of Academy of Management.

of what is possible (see Section 4.3). Whilst the original model of absorptive capacity separated the two phases of assimilation and transformation, Harvey et al. [7] use the concept of 'transformative learning' to combine them (Figure 5.2).

Finally, the organisation needs to actually use (*exploit*) the knowledge by implementing the recommendations in practice. As Section 5.5 explains, this phase depends on both resources and the competences of core staff.

Whilst absorptive capacity was originally developed from research in commercial organisations, it is at least as relevant to service organisations (such as health, education and social work) and the public sector as to the private sector [7]. Despite being described as 'one of the most important constructs to emerge in organisational research in recent decades' [9], absorptive capacity theory has only been applied in a handful of studies of evidence uptake in healthcare organisations. The ones I know about are described briefly in this section.

Back in 2005, Whitney Berta and her colleagues from Canada showed that differences between healthcare organisations in their success in implementing clinical practice guidelines were explained in significant part by differences in their absorptive capacity [10]. The same team has subsequently shown that this construct also explains differences in care homes' assimilation of innovative practices [11].

Gill Harvey and her team recently published a paper describing three organisational case studies of quality improvement initiatives [8]. Their findings were striking:

> The organisation with the highest [absorptive capacity] showed the quickest and most comprehensive performance improvement. Internal characteristics [of absorptive capacity] including strategic priorities, processes for managing information, communication and orientation to learning and development impacted on the organisation's ability to engage successfully with external stakeholders and make use of available knowledge. This enabled the organisation to thrive despite the challenging external environment. Lower levels of [absorptive capacity] appeared to delay or limit the improvement trajectory.

Absorptive capacity is closely related to the concept of team and organisational learning (discussed in Section 4.3) [12]. Indeed, Berta et al. [13] made the radical (but, I think, plausible and well-argued) suggestion that facilitation is an 'organisational meta-routine' that is central to the development and maintenance of absorptive capacity.

One of the reasons why absorptive capacity has been relatively little studied in healthcare organisations is that there is no validated methodology for measuring it quantitatively in such settings. A qualitative assessment of the multiple components of absorptive capacity is an essential prerequisite for developing a valid quantitative instrument, so the many qualitative studies of this construct in healthcare will (hopefully) inform such an exercise. Tessa Flattern and her team have used rich qualitative data followed by a rigorous quantitative phase to produce a validated scale of absorptive capacity in commercial organisations [14]; others are currently working on a comparable scale in the healthcare sector.

A related but broader construct for which we found strong empirical evidence in our 2004 review of diffusion of innovations is *receptive context*. An organisation that has the general features associated with receptivity to change (which includes both innovation – i.e. discontinuous change – and continuous quality improvement) will be better able to assimilate innovations [1].

Receptivity to change refers to willingness amongst an organisation's members to consider – individually and collectively – envisaged changes and to recognise their legitimacy. Receptivity as a process shapes and is shaped by the continuous sense-making and sense-giving activities conducted amongst various members of an organisation (see next section). It can be characterised as lying on a continuum from resistance to change at one extreme, through resigned passive acceptance, to enthusiastic endorsement at the other. The eight components of receptive context for change as originally developed by Andrew Pettigrew and colleagues back in 1992 (rephrased a little for clarity) are listed in Box 5.1.

Box 5.1 The eight components of receptive context for change

Within the organisation (covered in this chapter)

1 Visionary key people in critical posts leading change.
2 Good managerial and clinical relations.
3 Supportive organisational climate (one in which it's okay to take risks and try new things out).
4 Simplicity and clarity of goals and priorities.
5 Quality and coherence of 'policy' generated at a local level (including the presence of monitoring and feedback mechanisms to assess the change as it unfolds).

Beyond the organisation (covered in Chapters 9 and 10)

6 The role of intense environmental pressure in triggering periods of radical change.
7 The change agenda as interpreted locally, and how this agenda sits within the local health economy.
8 Development and management of a cooperative inter-organisational network.

Source: Pettigrew et al. [15]. *Reproduced with permission of Taylor & Francis.*

It will probably come as no surprise to find that change is more likely to happen if there is (in addition to the key features of absorptive capacity) strong leadership, clear strategic vision, good managerial relations, a climate conducive to experimentation and risk-taking (and especially psychological safety, which I define in Section 4.2 but which means, roughly translated, you won't get your head blown off when you raise a concern) and an effective monitoring and feedback system that is able to capture and process high-quality data.

Unsurprising they may be, but these key prerequisites are often forgotten when planning change initiatives in healthcare. Our book on diffusion of innovations reviewed numerous examples (now somewhat outdated) of where their omission explained failure of implementation [3].

5.4 Organisational readiness and the assimilation decision

An organisation may be amenable to innovation in general but not ready or willing to assimilate a particular innovation. Formal consideration of the innovation allows the organisation to move (or perhaps choose not to move) to a specific state of organisational readiness for that innovation. The key elements of organisational readiness for an innovation identified in our 2004 and 2010 reviews [1,5] are summarised in this section.

Tension for change
If staff in the organisation perceive that the present situation is intolerable, a potential innovation is more likely to be implemented successfully (strong direct evidence).

Innovation–system fit
An innovation that fits with the existing values, norms, strategies, goals, skill mix, supporting technologies and ways of working of the organisation is more likely to be assimilated and implemented successfully (strong indirect and moderate direct evidence).

Assessment of implications
If the implications of the innovation (including its knock-on effects) are fully assessed, anticipated and catered for, the innovation is more likely to be assimilated. In particular, job changes should be few and clear, appropriate training and support should be given and relevant documentation and augmentation (such as a helpdesk) should be provided for all technologies.

Support and advocacy
If supporters of the innovation outnumber, and are more strategically placed than, their opponents, the innovation is more likely to be assimilated and successfully implemented (see also social influence by opinion leaders and champions in Section 10.2).

Dedicated time and resources

If the innovation has a budget line and if resource allocation is both adequate and recurrent, the innovation is more likely to be assimilated.

Capacity to evaluate the innovation

If the organisation has tight systems and appropriate skills in place to monitor and evaluate the impact of the innovation, the innovation is more likely to be assimilated and sustained. Rapid, tight feedback enhances the organisation's ability to respond to this impact. In particular, measures must be in place to capture and respond to the various consequences of the innovation, including those that are:

- intended and predicted;
- unintended and predicted;
- unintended and unpredicted ('knock-on').

The process by which an organisation (or, sometimes, a department within an organisation) opts to assimilate an innovation is rarely a single, one-off decision. Rather, it typically involves a few weeks of what I would call 'argy-bargy'. Stuff happens not only in board meetings and committees but also outside of those formal structures. People have discussions in corridors; A seeks to bend the ear of B. Some people try out a version of the innovation; there may or may not be a formal pilot process.

During this period, the degree of fit (or lack of it) between the innovation and the organisational context becomes more evident – as do the various vested interests and a host of practical, material and technical considerations.

Jean-Louis Denis and colleagues [16] introduced the useful concept that an innovation always has a 'hard core' comprising features that define it (and without which it would not be the innovation) and a 'soft periphery' comprising things the organisation needs to have in place in order for the innovation to actually *work*. The soft periphery may include such things as physical space, broadband, new staff roles, a training programme, a technical support unit and so on. The assimilation phase can be thought of as a crucial opportunity to address 'soft periphery' elements.

Denis and colleagues [16] describe the process of negotiating the soft periphery as an ongoing exercise in micropolitics. Different stakeholders have different vested interests and different values. The risks and benefits of a complex innovation are not distributed evenly in an organisation or system: some will benefit, whilst others will experience negative consequences. The more the risks and benefits of the innovation map to the interests, values and power of the most powerful people in the organisation, the easier it is to build coalitions for the innovation's assimilation and subsequent routinisation.

Chapter 5

5.5 Implementation: balancing 'hard' and 'soft' efforts

Success in implementing and sustaining an organisational innovation in healthcare depends on many of the factors already covered in this chapter in relation to organisational readiness and the early stages of assimilation. In addition to readiness before adoption, additional elements are specifically associated with an innovation's successful implementation and routinisation (the defining feature of sustainability). Some of these measures are 'hard' (things you can measure objectively, count or draw in a diagram – such as budgets and tools); others are 'soft' (things less easily measured or represented – such as relationships and commitment). Both are crucial, of course.

SMART objectives

It may be a cliché that objectives should be specific, measurable, achievable, relevant and time-bound, but this is not a bad place to start when setting out to operationalise what you are actually going to do.

Staff involvement and commitment

Early and widespread involvement of staff at all levels – and, in particular, top management support and advocacy of the implementation process – enhances the success of implementation. See also Section 10.2 on the different kinds of social influence – especially peer and expert opinion leaders and champions.

Human resources

Successful implementation of an innovation in an organisation depends on the motivation, capacity and competence of individual practitioners. Appropriate training enhances the chances of effective implementation and of sustainability (moderate indirect and limited direct evidence).

Tools and techniques

The number of useful tools and techniques for implementing change in organisations now exceeds the capacity of any book to cover them. I have gathered some of my favourites into Appendix A.

Intra-organisational networks

Effective communication across internal structural (e.g. departmental) boundaries within an organisation enhances the success of implementation and the chances of sustainability. An explicitly narrative approach to intra-organisational networking (i.e. the purposive construction of a shared and emergent organisational story) can serve as a powerful cue to action (see next subsection).

Box 5.2 Seven elements of organisational sensemaking

- **Personal identity:** Organisational initiatives are closely tied up with people's sense of who they are.
- **Social context:** Sensemaking is a social activity in which stories are negotiated, retained and shared among organisational members.
- **Retrospection:** We make sense of things by looking back and crafting a story to explain what happened.
- **Ongoing nature of sensemaking:** People engage in a continuous stream of action; they simultaneously shape and react to the environments they face.
- **Plausibility:** Sensemaking requires plausible, believable stories. Indeed, people generally favour plausibility over accuracy, since people rarely agree on which 'facts' matter or what they are.
- **Salient clues:** People tend to elaborate tiny indicators into full-blown stories of 'success' or 'pulling together' – hence the importance of 'early wins'.
- **Enactment:** Sensemaking depends on continuous action and reflection on action by all of us (e.g. asking questions and probing to understand unfolding experience).

Source: Weick [17]. Reproduced with permission of SAGE Publications.

Chapter 5

Extra-organisational networks

These are often critical to the implementation process and are covered in more detail in Chapter 10. The greater the complexity of the implementation needed for a particular innovation, the greater the significance of the inter-organisational network to implementation success.

In relation to *intra*-organisational networking and dialogue, an important theoretical perspective has been developed by the US organisational sociologist Karl Weick. His construct of *organisational sensemaking* incorporates aspects of both absorptive capacity and receptivity to change (which are themselves closely related) [17]. I summarise the seven features of organisational sense-making in Box 5.2, and the main arguments in Weick's book on the subject in the next few paragraphs. There are parallels with Argyris and Schön's notion of organisational learning (which I have depicted as team learning), covered in Section 4.3.

When people are called upon to enact some innovation, they do so by trying to ascribe meaning to it. Organisational members are active 'framers', cognitively making sense of the events, processes, objects and issues that make up a complex innovation. A schema of a person's construction of reality provides the frame through which he or she recalls prior knowledge and interprets new information.

It inevitably is the case in innovation that the new idea, practice or object will be surprising; its adoption and use will clash with people's prevailing view of the organisation and what is or should be done in it. Unless encouraged to do otherwise, they will tend to retain the old schema (in which the innovation sits oddly) instead of discarding or modifying it. The result is cognitive inertia. The US management scholar Rosabeth Moss Kanter [18] has highlighted the political and sometimes frankly confrontational nature of innovation in organisations:

> *Innovation at its core … is replete with disputes caused by differences in perspectives among those touched by an innovation and the change it engenders.* (p. 231)

In other words, we should expect any change effort, and especially one that involves the discontinuous change of an innovation, to sit oddly within people's existing cognitive schemas. Weick's model of organisational sensemaking emphasises the evolutionary and action-based nature of the process. People don't make sense of innovation sitting in armchairs talking about it; they do stuff, and think about what they're doing. They engage in a continuous stream of action, which generates dissonant situations (ones that call for an explanation). They then retrospectively impose a cognitive schema on the situations they faced in order to make them sensible. These stories must be negotiated, since everyone's story is slightly different (we explain organisational action by imaginatively selecting elements out of the enacted environment to impugn causal relations between past events so as to deal with perceptions of dissonance and surprise).

Thus, sensemaking is a messy, conflict-ridden, continuous process that is less about 'facts' than about interpretations of a complex, shifting reality. The facilitation component of the PARIHS framework (see Section 4.3) might be seen as a relatively structured and systematic approach to helping this sensemaking process along. Incidentally, if you are grabbed (as I am) by Weick's take on sensemaking, you might like to look up his team's analysis of the Bristol Inquiry into the excess of cardiac deaths in paediatric cardiac surgery in a leading UK teaching hospital, which is presented as a pathological version of organisational sensemaking in which participants generated a collective narrative of 'success' despite what should have been seen as evidence of failure [19].

5.6 Routinisation and sustainability

A final theme I need to introduce in this chapter – and one that was identified as an emerging theme in our 2010 update of the diffusion of innovations review [5] – is that of *organisational routines*. If something is to become 'business as usual', it needs to be *routinised*. The routine is a key concept in

Box 5.3 Key features of organisational routines

1 Routines are recurrent, collective, interactive behaviour patterns.

2 Routines are specific (they have a history, a local context, and a particular set of relations) – hence, there is no such thing as universal best practice.

3 Routines coordinate (they work by enhancing interaction among participants).

4 Routines have two main purposes – cognition (knowledge of what to do) and governance (control).

5 By allowing actors to make many decisions at a subconscious level, routines conserve cognitive power for non-routine activities.

6 Routines store and pass on knowledge (especially tacit knowledge).

7 The knowledge for executing routines may be distributed (everyone has similar knowledge) or dispersed (everyone knows something different; overlaps are small).

8 Routines reduce uncertainty, and hence reduce the complexity of individual decisions.

9 Routines confer stability while containing the seeds of change (through the individual's response to feedback from previous iterations).

10 Routines change in a path dependent manner (depending on what has gone before).

11 Routines are triggered by actor-related factors (aspiration levels) and by external cues.

Source: Becker [21]. *Reproduced with permission of Oxford University Press.*

Chapter 5

organisation and management research; I described its relevance to healthcare innovation in a *BMJ* article in 2008 [20], which I summarise here.

An organisational routine is 'a repetitive, recognizable pattern of interdependent actions, involving multiple actors' [21]. Becker suggests that the routine may be the most fruitful unit of analysis when researching organisational change and sets out its defining characteristics (Box 5.3). One purpose of routines in organisations is to reduce uncertainty (and hence, cognitive dissonance and stress). On our first day in a new job, for example, we experience confusion because we do not 'know the ropes'. Work gradually becomes less stressful as we learn who to interact with, when, where and how. Another purpose is governance or control: a routine shapes and constrains the behaviour of people and makes some actions and processes impossible [21].

The development and delivery of effective routines depends on at least three things: structuring devices (time, space, documents, software, roles and responsibilities); people (on whose buy-in and mindful commitment a routine depends); and organisational learning (single-, double- and triple-loop – all described in Section 4.3). Collaborative work in organisations – of which contemporary healthcare is a prime example – is supported by the coming together of people at particular times and in particular places for an agreed set of tasks delivered through agreed roles and responsibilities, and with particular artefacts (documents, technologies) serving as focal points for such complex, collaborative tasks. This structuring process has been termed the 'grammar' of organisational life [22].

To routinise a new practice, object or way of working, we need to alter this fundamental grammar – and that is not an easy task. Indeed, it would seem that routines are the root of organisational inertia. Yet, as Martha Feldman has argued in a landmark theoretical paper, it is – paradoxically – in routines that the scope for organisational change and innovation lies. As she puts it:

> Routines are performed by people who think and feel and care. Their reactions are situated in institutional, organisational and personal contexts. Their actions are motivated by will and intention. All of these forces influence the enactment of organisational routines and create in them a tremendous potential for change. [23]

Feldman's point is, every time a routine is enacted, it is done slightly differently. Human agents can perform the routine half-heartedly and/or in a way that leads to its eventual attrition – or they can, every time the routine is enacted, make their contribution sharper and better, thus inspiring others to enhance their own contribution. People can help improve the use of the artefacts and other structures that support the routine – or they can subvert the use of those artefacts (e.g. by 'forgetting' passwords or turning up late). And team leaders can support the shaping of routines – either positively by praising and resourcing staff who enact them well, or negatively by failing to notice or reward these efforts.

Much more could be said about the research literature on routinisation in healthcare, but this chapter is already long enough. If you are interested in how the study of routines can shed new light on topics such as patient safety, see my team's study (led by Deborah Swinglehurst) of how healthcare receptionists ensure safety in repeat prescribing routines [24] or the accounts by Jie Mein Goh [25] and Laurie Novak [26] of adaptive implementation of information technology in healthcare settings. There is more (tangentially) on routinisation of innovations in Section 8.4, where I consider why clinicians are so often resistant to the introduction of new technologies.

In Appendix A, I introduce the tool of process mapping – which may get you started, but is not itself a way of surfacing the kind of detail needed for an academic analysis of organisational routines. I also introduce the NHS Institute for Innovation and Improvement (NHS III) Sustainability Model, which is believed by some to be a tool for improving the sustainability of service-level innovations. As I point out, this tool contains some helpful things to think about when seeking to implement such innovations, but I am unconvinced that it really gets to the bottom of the sustainability question.

5.7 Ten tips for promoting organisational innovation

If you do not have a senior role in your organisation, you may not be able to effect major change in the way the organisation operates. That does not mean there are no options open to you, but it may mean that your menu of options is limited to smaller-scale activities at an interpersonal (Chapter 3) or team (Chapter 4) level.

However, if you are the chief executive of your organisation – or a clinical director, departmental manager, non-executive director or similar – you should be thinking strategically about how to build your organisation's capacity to innovate (Tips 1 to 5) and how to help it evaluate, introduce and embed particular evidence-based innovations (Tips 6 to 10). These tips are based on my own work and that of others cited earlier in this chapter; they also draw eclectically on Rosabeth Moss Kanter's 'rules for stifling innovation' (and, conversely, ways of avoiding doing so), published a few years ago in her book, *The Change Masters* [27].

To build your organisation's general capacity to innovate
1. Do as much as you can to flatten and decentralise
the management structure
As noted in Section 5.2, the evidence from business and management studies is strong and consistent: introducing anything new is inherently difficult when every decision has to be passed up a complex hierarchy for signing off. Far better to appoint good people, then leave them to lead their teams and make frontline decisions. Innovation may well follow. One important aspect of a decentralised management structure is distributed leadership (see Section 4.2). Does everyone in the organisation think that *you* are the leader on every project – or is there a sense that most projects are collaborative endeavours in which many people, right across the organisation and often beyond it, need to display leadership and vision? Evidence suggests you'll achieve faster and more enduring innovation if the latter holds true.

2. Create and distribute slack resources
'Slack resources' means spare money, time, people and space that innovators can draw upon to support new projects (see Section 5.2). This is not about senior managers deciding to fund project X but about resources being available to support good ideas whenever and wherever they emerge right across the organisation. And good ideas are as likely to come from a group of student nurses as they are from the Senior Executive Committee. Sometimes,

the amount of money needed is tiny (photocopying costs, refreshments for a meeting, a few hours' back-fill of a clinician's time), but the project will not get to first base if these resources are not forthcoming.

3. Foster a risk-taking climate

I explained in Section 5.3 that innovation is more likely to happen in organisations in which it is seen as acceptable (indeed, desirable) to take risks. If you punish someone because they pursued an idea that did not work out, and especially if you frame the project's failure as the fault of one or two aspiring innovators, the organisational grapevine will soon spread the message that experimenting in good faith gets you into trouble. On the other hand, if you publicly thank the staff member (or group) who 'had a go' and help staff draw out positive lessons from a 'failed' project, the message will soon circulate that the boss has a mature and creative approach to risk. Remember: commend people's efforts in public and criticise individuals (if you must) in private.

4. Nurture relationships

As noted in Section 5.3, case study after case study has identified 'good clinical and managerial relationships' as key to successful innovation. How do you support the building of such relationships? Providing space and opportunity for people to meet and talk would be a good start. Avoid language that assumes (and perpetuates) an 'us and them' culture. Make sure that as far as possible, teams and working groups include both clinicians and managers. This is how trust, friendships and social networks develop – and it is these human linkages, not the formal organisational chart, that form the scaffolding for effective change.

5. Build absorptive capacity

As I explained in Section 5.3, absorptive capacity is an organisation's ability to acquire, assimilate, transform and exploit knowledge. Work is ongoing to develop formal metrics of absorptive capacity in healthcare organisations. Until these are available, I suggest you use the following questions to get a handle on your organisation's absorptive capacity:

- Does our organisation already have a stock of internal knowledge on key topic areas (people who know stuff and resources that people can use to look up knowledge)?
- Do we have the infrastructure to bring in more knowledge on these topics – such as high-quality systems for capturing and managing relevant data?
- Do we invest in measures to seek out and capture knowledge – for example, by sending staff on courses, conducting horizon-scanning work and assigning dedicated knowledge roles?

- When we send staff on courses, do we routinely create opportunities for them to consolidate their learning and work out how to apply it to their own work?
- Do we routinely create opportunities for staff to come together to share their learning (from external courses or internal audits) with others, and discuss its implications for how care is delivered? To put that another way, is *transformative learning* (in which the dry, abstract knowledge from continuing professional development courses is discussed and reframed to make it meaningful to real-life practice) actively supported?
- When individual and team learning suggests that current practice should change, is our organisation good at putting measures in place to implement and evaluate changes? Do we allocate time to such activity – and do we reward staff for being creative in this regard?

To support the introduction of a specific innovation
6. Systematically assess whether the innovation is right for the organisation

Before you take your organisation headlong into an initiative that will have a major impact on staff and patients, consider carefully whether this innovation is the right step for this organisation, at this time. Look back at Section 5.4. Is there tension for change? Does the innovation 'fit' the organisation (in terms of your long-term mission, medium-term goals, values, priorities, existing infrastructure and consideration of competing tasks and issues)? What are the implications for the organisation as a whole and for particular teams, departments and individuals? Who will need (re-)training, when and by whom? To what extent will the innovation be supported by key staff – and what 'wrecking power' is held by its opponents? Can a budget line be found for supporting its introduction – and for evaluating its impact?

7. Attend judiciously to project management

To the extent that introducing the innovation is a 'project' (as opposed to a more nebulous entity like 'changing culture'), there are some basic rules for improving its chances of success. Ensure that the goals of the project are simple, clear and (if possible) agreed amongst key stakeholders. Convert these to SMART objectives (see Section 5.5), with a named individual responsible for delivering on each (and reporting to another named individual or committee). Select and apply key metrics for monitoring progress and feeding back (and reflecting on) real-time data. Don't try to measure everything or the project will be weighted down by its own evaluation (Appendix A may give you some ideas on what to measure and how). Train and develop staff, and provide helpdesk support for new technologies and technology-dependent processes.

Having said that, don't forget that one of Kanter's rules for stifling innovation is to hold people rigidly to project plans and timescales (count everything that can be counted, insist that all procedures be followed to the letter, and so on) [27]. Use your intuition and judgement to decide when to be in 'project management' mode and when to step back from bean-counting and clock-watching.

8. Value and support organisational sensemaking

The 'soft' aspects of introducing innovation (see Section 5.5) are as important as the 'hard'. We all know we have to get people on board – but not everyone realises that one way to do this is by inviting widespread discussion in which dissenters can voice their concerns openly. You may well find that such discussions (sometimes referred to as 'town meetings') surface legitimate concerns from frontline staff – but they also allow the supporters of the innovation to articulate the arguments in its favour. As Kanter emphasises, don't make the mistake of restricting discussion of strategies and plans to a small inner circle of senior staff and announcing decisions in full-blown form. Far better to consult on an outline, solicit and take note of feedback, and thank the organisational members for helping to shape a plan that (hopefully) now has a high chance of working. Encourage and support the development of informal, lateral networks across the organisation – either virtually or face to face. (Through such networks, people will exchange the countless big and small ideas, resources, tips and offers of support that make it possible to convert an abstract blueprint into an enacted, sustainable change.)

9. Study organisational routines and the interactions between them

Often, a new project does pretty well whilst it is considered in isolation from the mundane reality of organisational life – when it's just So-and-So's 'pet project'. But when So-and-So leaves, or gets distracted into something else, the original initiative is likely to fade away rapidly. As I emphasised in Section 5.6, in order to be sustained, a new practice must be routinised (i.e. made business as usual) – and the routine must interface smoothly with other (existing) routines. In Appendix A, I introduce the technique of process mapping to tease out the key steps in a routine. But don't forget Feldman's observation that routines are implemented by human actors who (to a greater or lesser extent) think and feel and care. The human dimension (who is doing the task, how much they care about it, how much it is valued) is at least as important as the abstracted map of what needs to be done.

10. Encourage links beyond the organisation

Introducing innovation is a pragmatic, contingent and dynamic task. Whilst the evidence may be clear and abstract (expressed, for example, in terms of numbers needed to treat or incremental cost-effectiveness ratios), the *implementation* of that evidence necessarily happens in the down-and-dirty of organisational work. You're going to need 'lines to take' (with key staff groups), job descriptions, agendas for meetings, metrics, reporting structures, informal workarounds, 'plan Bs' and so on. A good way of getting going – and making progress – with these practical measures is to get key frontline staff to link up with their counterparts in other organisations who are introducing the same innovation – either virtually or at face-to-face conferences and workshops. Networks (of various kinds) are so important in the innovation process that I have dedicated an entire chapter to them (Chapter 10). My point here is that networking beyond the organisation is something that organisational leaders should be actively encouraging and supporting.

References

1. Greenhalgh, T., Robert, G., Macfarlane, F., Bate, P., & Kyriakidou, O. (2004). Diffusion of innovations in service organizations: systematic review and recommendations. *The Milbank Quarterly*, **82**(4), 581–629.

2. Greenhalgh, T., Robert, G., Macfarlane, F., Bate, P., Kyriakidou, O., & Peacock, R. (2005). Storylines of research in diffusion of innovation: a meta-narrative approach to systematic review. *Social Science & Medicine (1982)*, **61**(2), 417–430.

3. Greenhalgh, T., Robert, G., Bate, P., Kyriakidou, O., & Macfarlane, F. (2005). *Diffusion of Innovations in Health Service Organisations: A Systematic Literature Review*. Oxford, Blackwells.

4. Wong, G., Greenhalgh, T., Westhorp, G., Buckingham, J., & Pawson, R. (2013). RAMESES publication standards: meta-narrative reviews. *BMC Medicine*, **11**, 20.

5. Robert, G., Greenhalgh, T., MacFarlane, F., & Peacock, R. (2010). Adopting and assimilating new non-pharmaceutical technologies into health care: a systematic review. *Journal of Health Services Research & Policy*, **15**(4), 243–250.

6. Zahra, S.A., & George, G. (2002). Absorptive capacity: a review, reconceptualization, and extension. *Academy of Management Review*, **27**(2), 185–203.

7. Harvey, G., Skelcher, C., Spencer, E., Jas, P., & Walshe, K. (2010). Absorptive capacity in a non-market environment: a knowledge-based approach to analysing the performance of sector organizations. *Public Management Review*, **12**(1), 77–97.

8. Harvey, G., Jas, P., & Walshe, K. (2014). Analysing organisational context: case studies on the contribution of absorptive capacity theory to understanding inter-organisational variation in performance improvement. *BMJ Quality & Safety*, **24**(1), 48–55.

9. Lane, P.J., Koka, B.R., & Pathak, S. (2006). The reification of absorptive capacity: a critical review and rejuvenation of the construct. *Academy of Management Review*, **31**(4), 833–863.

10. Berta, W., Teare, G.F., Gilbart, E., Ginsburg, L.S., Lemieux-Charles, L., Davis, D., & Rappolt, S. (2005). The contingencies of organizational learning in long-term care: factors that affect innovation adoption. *Health Care Management Review*, **30**(4), 282–292.

Chapter 5

11. Berta, W., Teare, G.F., Gilbart, E., Ginsburg, L.S., Lemieux-Charles, L., Davis, D., & Rappolt, S. (2010). Spanning the know-do gap: understanding knowledge application and capacity in long-term care homes. *Social Science & Medicine*, **70**(9), 1326–1334.

12. Argyris, C., & Schön, D. (1978). *Organizational Learning: A Theory of Action Perspective*. Reading, MA, Addision-Wesley.

13. Berta, W., Cranley, L., Dearing, J.W., Dogherty, E.J., Squires, J.E., & Estabrooks, C.A. (2015). Why (we think) facilitation works: insights from organizational learning theory. *Implementation Science*, **10**(1), 141.

14. Flatten, T.C., Engelen, A., Zahra, S.A., & Brettel, M. (2011). A measure of absorptive capacity: Scale development and validation. *European Management Journal*, **29**(2), 98–116.

15. Pettigrew, A., Ferlie, E., & McKee, L. (1992). Shaping strategic change – the case of the NHS in the 1980s. *Public Money & Management*, **12**(3), 27–31.

16. Denis, J.-L., Hébert, Y., Langley, A., Lozeau, D., & Trottier, L.-H. (2002). Explaining diffusion patterns for complex health care innovations. *Health Care Management Review*, **27**(3), 60–73.

17. Weick, K.E. (1995). *Sensemaking in Organizations (Foundations for Organizational Science)*. Thousands Oaks, CA, Sage Publications.

18. Kanter, R.M. (1990). *When Giants Learn to Dance*. London, Simon and Schuster.

19. Weick, K.E., Sutcliffe, K.M., & Obstfeld, D. (2005). Organizing and the process of sensemaking. *Organization Science*, **16**(4), 409–421.

20. Greenhalgh, T. (2008). Role of routines in collaborative work in healthcare organisations. *BMJ*, **337**, a2448.

21. Becker, M.C. (2004). Organizational routines: a review of the literature. *Industrial and Corporate Change*, **13**(4), 643–678.

22. Pentland, B.T. (1995). Grammatical models of organizational processes. *Organization Science*, **6**(5), 541–556.

23. Feldman, M.S. (2000). Organizational routines as a source of continuous change. *Organization Science*, **11**(6), 611–629.

24. Swinglehurst, D., Greenhalgh, T., Russell, J., & Myall, M. (2011). Receptionist input to quality and safety in repeat prescribing in UK general practice: ethnographic case study. *BMJ*, **343**, d6788.

25. Goh, J.M., Gao, G., & Agarwal, R. (2011). Evolving work routines: adaptive routinization of information technology in healthcare. *Information Systems Research*, **22**(3), 565–585.

26. Novak, L., Brooks, J., Gadd, C., Anders, S., & Lorenzi, N. (2012). Mediating the intersections of organizational routines during the introduction of a health IT system. *European Journal of Information Systems*, **21**(5), 552–569.

27. Kanter, R.M. (1984). *The Change Masters*. New York, Simon and Schuster.

Chapter 6 **Citizens**

6.1 Citizens, the public, lay people – who are they (we)?

There is much overlap between 'citizens' (this chapter) and 'patients' (Chapter 7). We are all both at times, sometimes concurrently. So the division into two separate chapters is somewhat artificial (but necessary, since there is too much to say for one chapter). Citizens and patients are people, of course, so everything I said in Chapter 3 about the psychology of human behaviour also applies (broadly speaking) to both of them.

The terms 'public', 'lay people', 'consumers', 'citizens', 'patients', 'service users' and 'research participants' are not interchangeable (although it has to be said, those who make it their business to emphasise the fine distinctions between these terms can be a bit pedantic at times). Table 6.1 offers some definitions. These are my own, but based on my reading of the wider literature referenced in this chapter. Note the bottom row: the term 'subject' is obsolete; people who take part in research should be called 'participants'. When I road-tested a draft of Table 6.1 on my Twitter followers, I sparked a heated debate about which terms should be in the table and how they should be defined. The Healthtalk research team (www.healthtalk.org) asked their lay partners, and found that different people wanted to go by different names (although 'consumer' was almost universally disliked). So confusion reigns.

This chapter focuses on the involvement of lay people when they are thinking generally about research and evidence, rather than when making decisions that relate to their own illness and healthcare in the here and now. It covers five main topics: the different degrees of lay involvement in research (Section 6.2); how we might design research studies to make them more patient-centred (Section 6.3); how we might involve lay people (including patients) more closely in research (Section 6.4); and how to communicate science to the lay public (Section 6.5). The next chapter considers how to apply the evidence-based healthcare (EBHC) agenda with patients when they are directly receiving healthcare, either in the clinical consultation or in the

How to Implement Evidence-Based Healthcare, First Edition. Trisha Greenhalgh.
© 2018 John Wiley & Sons Ltd. Published 2018 by John Wiley & Sons Ltd.

Table 6.1 Some definitions of terms for lay people when involved in research or clinical governance.

Term	Definition	When to use this term
Public	All of us, especially in a defined country or geographical region	When talking about accountability to the public (e.g. whether something is a good use of people's taxes)
Citizen	Almost the singular of 'the public' (except that some people, e.g. refugees, lack full citizenship status)	When looking for someone to represent the public perspective, whose primary orientation is to the public good
Lay people	People who do not have expertise or training in a particular field but who are nevertheless affected by it	When looking for the voice of ordinary experience and/or common sense (usually to balance a group otherwise composed of experts)
Patients	People who are seeking or receiving healthcare	When looking for expertise in what it means to be ill and/or receive care (may be called 'experts by experience')
Clients	People who are seeking or receiving social care and (sometimes) care from allied professions or therapists	As with patients, but in the social care/allied health field
Carers	People who help another individual look after themselves and access services	When looking for expertise in what it means to care for someone and/or on the wider impact of illness on the family
Service users	People who use or seek to use a health or social service (including patients, carers, parents)	When looking for the user experience of accessing and using services
Advocates	People who speak (and who have a mandate to speak) for a particular vulnerable person or group	When seeking the perspective of an individual or group who finds it awkward or impossible to provide that perspective themselves
Consumers	People who make choices (and – usually, although not always – pay for them)	Where information is being produced to inform a choice (e.g. by patients, service users or their families and carers)
Research participants	Humans who take part in research	When undertaking research or seeking the perspective of those who take part in research
Subjects	Animals on whom research is done	Not to be used when referring to humans, except in relation to the UK Data Protection Act ('data subject')

process of managing their illness in daily life. To those who say this book is supposed to be about implementing the findings of high-quality research, not about the research process, I would remind you that the best way to ensure that something is accepted and implemented is to involve the intended users in its design.

In this of all chapters, please don't expect a definitive set of mechanical formulae and checklists. Whilst such algorithmic approaches to citizen and lay involvement certainly exist, I don't believe in them and have not, in general, referenced them. I acknowledge the important work of INVOLVE on patient and public involvement in research [1], although I do not always fully agree with how they frame the issues. The UK Health Research Agency (a statutory body established to promote public involvement in research) also has an excellent website of resources (http://www.hra.nhs.uk/resources/public-involvement-research/).

Lay involvement in the research process is viewed as an ethical imperative in its own right [2,3]; as a means to making research more efficient and more implementable [4]; and as a way to widen the scope of research to embrace the subjective, experiential knowledge of the patient as well as the objective knowledge of clinical measurement [5]. It is said to improve the process of research (e.g. representativeness, recruitment and retention in trials) [1], reduce waste [6,7] and increase impact (e.g. acceptance by patients and clinicians) [8], although some authors have cautioned against an overly instrumental view of lay involvement (e.g. doing it *in order to* increase recruitment, rather than because you respect the right of patients and the public to be involved) [2].

Lay input to health technology appraisal (the assessment of research evidence to produce guidance and recommendations – such as the work of the National Institute for Health and Care Excellence (NICE) in the United Kingdom) 'provides meaning to the data, bringing the numbers to life' [9].

Figure 6.1, which is adapted from a figure initially produced by Jonathan Boote and colleagues [4], offers a rough taxonomy of how citizens and lay people, either individually or as members of local, national or international groups, might become involved in the research process or the implementation of research.

Patients and other lay people who take on the role of 'representative' on research steering groups or service improvement activities are what epidemiologists would call a self-selecting (and hence statistically biased) sample. Barnes et al. [10] have proposed three types of lay representativeness: (i) 'democratic' representativeness, where the individual is elected by his or her peers (and thus has a formal mandate to speak on their behalf); (ii) 'statistical' representativeness, where the individual is judged to be mathematically representative of a particular group (e.g. because they have neither a very

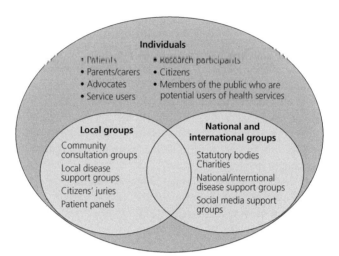

Figure 6.1 Taxonomy of lay and public involvement. *Source:* Boote et al. [4]. Reproduced with permission of Elsevier.

mild nor a very severe form of a condition); and (iii) 'typical' representativeness, where the indiviudal is considered to share key characteristics and/or experiences with the group represented (e.g. a user of dialysis services).

As Table 6.1 indicates, lay people are often defined in terms of what they are not (not researchers, not clinicians, not knowledgeable, not socialised into organisational culture, not on the payroll and so on) rather than in terms of the positive aspects of who they are or what they might bring [11]. It is assumed (perhaps incorrectly) that such people will therefore bring a dose of 'ordinariness' or common sense to a public consultation or to a group that is otherwise composed of researchers, clinicians or other in-house members. This, of course, is a naïve framing of the complex role of the 'lay member' in any group.

I will not resolve this tension in this chapter (it is, arguably, unresolvable), but I will warn you to keep a healthy scepticism about the term 'lay' as you consider the evidence base on citizen and patient involvement in either the conduct of research (this chapter) or its implementation in service improvement (Section 7.4).

6.2 Lay involvement in research: how much and on whose terms?

Involvement is not the same as 'democratic partnership'. In my view, tokenism in relation to lay involvement in research is rife. Inviting your pet patient (who probably shares your social class, ethnic background and perhaps age and gender as well) to sit on the steering group of your research study might tick the PPI (patient and public involvement) box on the grant application form, but it would sit close to the bottom of any hierarchy of genuine involvement. You can and should do better.

Before we get into the question of 'How much and on whose terms?', we need to be clear that citizen involvement is not merely a technical process. Rather, it is based on values. In its guidance, a team based at the Universities of Lancaster, Liverpool and Exeter, led by Jennie Popay, identified three different kinds of value [12]:

1. values relating to interpersonal relationships (i.e. relationships between researchers and the public based on respect and trust);
2. values relating to organisational issues (i.e. public involvement leading to research of greater quality and relevance to the healthcare system);
3. societal values (i.e. accountability and transparency of the research processes to the wider community).

These authors suggest that the first step in developing an approach to citizen involvement in research is to make the different values explicit and to acknowledge that different stakeholders will be seeking to undertake (or, indeed, block) citizen involvement for different underlying reasons.

Values often clash. For example, researchers adhere strongly to scientific values about what kinds of research design are the best to use in different circumstances. These values sometimes conflict with citizen values about priorities and equity.

I was once involved in a systematic review of school feeding programmes in low-income settings [13]. One paper in our sample described a study in which researchers sought to randomise the children in school classes to receiving or not receiving a food supplement (this would have controlled for the effects of the teacher). Both the teachers and the parents, however, were much more concerned about the ethics (and practicalities) of withholding food from one half of a class of severely undernourished children! To the great credit of the research team, the study was changed to a before-and-after design – scientifically less robust but (I believe) more justified in the circumstances.

For an authoritative narrative review of values in citizen involvement in research, see a paper by Gradinger et al. [14].

Various approaches seek to measure power sharing in collaborative programmes. One-dimensional scales of citizen involvement – the most famous example being Sherry Arnstein's Ladder of Participation, which climbs from 'manipulation' (in which citizens are coerced) to 'citizen control' (in which citizens set the agenda) [15] – have been largely superseded in the academic literature by more qualitative taxonomies that seek to capture *who* is participating, in *what* and for *whose* benefit [16,17].

My favourite scale of lay involvement in research (because it is simple, intuitive and easy to apply) comes from Sarah White, who writes in the community-based participatory research literature. She distinguishes *nominal* involvement of citizens (undertaken to confer legitimacy on a project), *instrumental* involvement (to improve the project's delivery and/or efficiency), *representative* involvement (to avoid creating dependency) and *transformative* involvement (to enable citizens to influence their own destiny) [18]. The National Institute for Health Research (NIHR) offers a similar taxonomy: consultative (in which researchers consult patients or lay people, perhaps individually), collaborative (some sort of partnership with a user group) and user-driven (in which users set the agenda and researchers respond) [19].

Sandy Oliver and colleagues have proposed two dimensions for thinking about lay involvement in research [3]. The first dimension is effectively a four-rung ladder of participation for lay people consisting of minimal, consultation, collaboration and lay control; the second is the amount of effort the researchers put in to engaging with the lay agenda, on a scale of minimal or nil, responding to lay action (e.g. a complaint or lobbying), inviting individual lay people to be represented and inviting lay groups. I have used this simple grading system in Figure 6.2, where I illustrate various scenarios of power-sharing and relationships with researchers. Note that power-sharing in a 'responsive' mode with lay groups may lead to the most vocal single-issue campaigns tending to dominate the agenda.

In the field of community-based participatory research (done locally and with the goal of benefiting local people, as well as adding to the wider knowledge base), additional dimensions of lay involvement include the extent to which research designs are culturally and logistically *appropriate*; the extent of measures to develop *capacity and capability* in the community partner (e.g. Are any community members trained in research skills?); how and to what extent *conflicts* are managed; and the extent to which *mutual trust* builds over time [20].

In sum, the principle of public, patient and lay involvement in research is widely accepted and – if done well – will almost certainly make the findings more widely accepted and more easily implemented. But the practicalities are no small hurdle. If you are planning the patient and public involvement section of a research study, I strongly encourage you to explore the topic in more depth via the sources referenced at the end of this chapter. One to note is Popay and team's Public Involvement Impact Assessment Framework – a structured approach to evaluating the impact of citizen involvement initiatives [12]. The framework is described briefly in Appendix A.

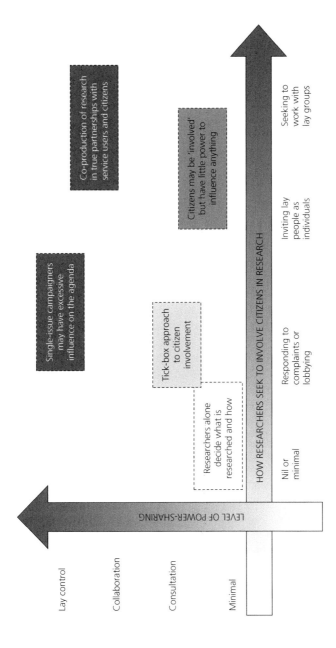

Figure 6.2 Citizen involvement in research – a two-dimensional model. *Source:* Based on Oliver et al.'s original taxonomy [3].

6.3 'We ask the questions': moving beyond a researcher-focused EBHC

The first step towards generating the kinds of research that patients will find relevant (and want to see implemented) is to ask the kinds of question that matter to patients. We are all patients from time to time, of course – and it's when we are the one lying in the hospital bed or sitting nervously in the waiting room that we realise that the 'evidence' on which our management is based has somehow missed the mark. Let me give you some examples from my own experience (one as a researcher and one as a patient).

Many years ago, I was asked to co-chair a national exercise to set future research priorities in diabetes. We set up a series of focus groups. Some consisted of researchers and clinicians and some of patients and carers, and we ran them in that order. The professionals identified a number of priorities – including studies into behaviour change (by which they meant, how to change patients' behaviour so they followed healthier lifestyles and took their medication more consistently). When we proposed the idea of 'behaviour change' research to the patient focus groups, they were very enthusiastic – but only because they thought we meant research to change the behaviour of *doctors* (to make them less judgemental, less naïve about the realities of living with diabetes and less paternalistic). In the end, we recommended research into both kinds of 'behaviour change'.

A few years back, I was diagnosed with osteopenia and advised to take the bone-strengthening drug alendronate at a dose of 70 mg once a week. Both the benefits and the side effects were fully explained to me: the drug had a high chance of preventing me developing crippling osteoporosis (as my grandmother and mother had done before me), but at the cost of a host of gastrointestinal symptoms (discomfort, collywobbles, diarrhoea, you name it) and a more serious but less likely risk that a tablet might actually perforate my oesophagus on the way down. I had to take the tablet standing up, wash it down with a long swig of water and then cross my fingers that it would not burn a hole in my mucosa on its journey to my stomach.

Being a good patient, I began by taking my alendronate faithfully every Sunday morning – and I hated it. Because the collywobbles were worse when I bent over, it messed up the Sunday morning bike ride that my husband and I had been doing for the previous 30 years. I shifted my drug day to Saturdays – and got caught short in the supermarket. I shifted to Mondays – and found myself sitting in committees or student supervisions with my tummy protesting loudly.

I did not want to take alendronate every week. But I did not want to get osteoporosis, either. So I formulated (subconsciously at first) a question in my head: 'What is the minimum amount of alendronate I need to take in order to get the benefits? Perhaps once a fortnight or once a month would be okay.'

I then searched Medline and found abundant evidence that many patients discontinue alendronate because of side effects [21], and one study from China (whose generalisability to a Caucasian population is questionable) suggesting that fortnightly dosing was as effective as weekly [22]. Nobody appeared to have tested once-a-month dosing. I had identified an important knowledge gap.

Pharmaceutical companies are unlikely to prioritise research studies that could end up reducing their sales. But the government-funded UK Health Technology Assessment (HTA) programme is keen to develop the evidence base for reducing unnecessary prescribing. As a general principle, *every* patient should be on the minimum effective dose of the fewest drugs possible. On the advice of my colleague James Raftery, I submitted a request to the HTA's 'Identifying Topics for Research' website (www.nets.nihr.ac.uk/identifying-research), arguing from the patient perspective that I'd like to know how much I could 'down-titrate' my dosage. I did not actually use the word 'down-titrate', but that is how my question was rephrased for the research community. My idea was considered by a panel and recommended for priority funding in 2016. In the next edition of this book, I will tell you whether anyone took up the idea and started a trial. If they do, I have offered to be a patient adviser on the study steering group.

I would not want to second-guess the findings of yet-to-be-conducted research on this particular topic, but I hope you can see that inviting patients to set at least part of the research agenda could lead to findings that improve effectiveness *and* reduce waste in research (in the alendronate example, by seeking to reduce the risk of patients discontinuing their medication and optimising the amount of drug given to each patient) [6,7].

Not many patients will have the confidence and the wherewithal to start suggesting ideas for new clinical trials direct to the government. The HTA's 'Suggestions' website, whilst welcome, is therefore only a partial solution to the lack of patient input to research design. Patient charities (MIND, Diabetes UK, Arthritis Research and so on) undertake extensive consultation with their members and feed the findings into research priority-setting.

Another important initiative is the James Lind Alliance (JLA, www.jla.nihr.ac.uk), a non-profit-making UK initiative established in 2004, whose mission is to establish 'Priority Setting Partnerships' of patients, carers and healthcare professionals with a democratic ethos (everyone's perspective counts) so as to inform the work of both academic researchers and industry. JLA groups identify unanswered questions about treatment (which they refer to as 'uncertainties') and work jointly with patients and professionals to prioritise these into a 'top ten' list of topics that can be presented to potential research funders.

The rationale behind the JLA is that patients and carers bring expertise on the lived experience whilst professionals bring a more scientific kind of

Chapter 6

expertise; the best research questions will emerge from productive dialogue between these experts. For an example of JLA work in Parkinson's disease, see a paper by Deane et al. [23].

Worthy though its goals are, the JLA has recently been criticised by patient groups for its allegedly tokenistic involvement of patients (patients felt that they were accused, for example, of suggesting the 'wrong kind of questions') [24]. Perhaps we should all acknowledge that the science (and art) of involving patients in research priority-setting is in its infancy and there are many unanswered questions about the process itself. I was pleased to see that at least one group has published a protocol for an in-depth qualitative study on this topic [25].

Another dimension of patient involvement in research is establishing outcome measures that matter to patients. We are always told, 'Treat the patient, not the blood test/X-ray result/risk factor etc.' – but what exactly *should* we be measuring to define success in different conditions? In heart failure, for example, researchers have tended to measure success in terms of increased survival and reduced hospital admission (both of which can sometimes be achieved by 'up-titration' of medication), whereas in my own experience, patients with heart failure may prefer to trade a few weeks' survival advantage for better quality of life (more likely if medication is *not* up-titrated to optimise a blood test result!).

The science of patient-reported outcome measures (PROMs) aims to develop 'standardised, validated questionnaires that are completed by patients to measure their perceptions of their own functional status and wellbeing' [26] using a combination of in-depth qualitative research and systematic surveys of people who have the condition being researched. Factoring in the patient perspective in trial design is an important step forward. But PROMs and similar instruments – which effectively give us patients' priorities 'on average' – can never fully capture the situated, fluctuating granularity of what matters most to a particular patient or carer at a particular point in the illness journey (including why the person has or has not consulted the clinician at a key decision point).

In sum, involving patients and citizens in setting research priorities and designing research studies is an important contribution to reducing research waste and improving the chances of research findings being successfully implemented – but it is not a straightforward process. I look forward to seeing the results of ongoing research into this topic.

6.4 Conducting research with (as opposed to on) patients

Even when patients have helped set the questions and define the outcome measures for research, researchers generally need reminding of the patient perspective whilst actually planning, doing and writing up research studies.

All the major health research funders in the United Kingdom now require patients and citizens to be involved in what is known as research governance – that is, the overseeing of good practice when a piece of research is undertaken.

Nathan Shippee and colleagues have undertaken a systematic review of research studies on patient involvement in research, based on a traditional, linear model of the research journey from preparation to execution and then translation [27]. In this model, components of patient and lay involvement consist of:

- how to initiate the study (i.e. recruitment of patients and service users);
- how to develop reciprocal relationships (i.e. ensure that patient involvement is democratic rather than tokenistic and that lay members of panels feel able to speak out);
- co-learning (things that patients need to learn about research and things that researchers need to learn about patients in this context);
- the importance of assessing progress and feeding back to improve the success of the initiative.

I am a little uncomfortable with the way Shippee and colleagues framed their review (and that, of course, partly reflects the way the underpinning primary research studies had been framed). It seems to me to be (unwittingly) somewhat researcher-centred ('How can we get more patients involved with *our* research?' as opposed to 'How can we find out what patients and service user groups are already doing and adapt our research radically to help them achieve their goals?'). But I should not be too hard on these authors because I, too, wear a researcher hat most of the time and spend long hours trying to recruit, engage and develop relationships with patients for *my* research!

A radically different approach to involving patients and citizens in research is known as *co-creation* or *co-design*. The concept of knowledge translation or 'getting research into practice' is predicated on the assumption that research knowledge is created by university-based (or industry-based) scientists and *then* packaged and processed in a way that makes it accessible to non-scientists. Yet not all research conforms to this linear sequence.

In 1994, a book entitled *The New Production of Knowledge* introduced a new taxonomy: 'Mode 1 scientific discovery' and 'Mode 2 knowledge production' [28]. Mode 1 refers to the conventional model of university-based research, which is then 'translated'. Gibbons et al. [29] describe this mode as 'hegemonic' (i.e. relating to domination) and driven by closed hierarchies of scientists and their universities, implicitly at the expense of non-academic stakeholders. Mode 2 knowledge, in contrast, is 'socially distributed, application-oriented, trans-disciplinary and subject to multiple accountabilities' [29].

Such knowledge is generated largely outside the university, and often at the very site where it will be applied. University scientists come together with frontline clinicians, community members, policymakers, citizens and others to identify and prioritise questions, develop research methodologies, collect and analyse data and implement findings. There are many players, many experts (of different kinds) and an evolving collective view (although rarely a consensus) on what the questions and challenges are.

Let me give you an example. I recently sat on a commission to address health inequalities in the region where I work. I was representing the university; other people who sat on the group (or who were invited to provide evidence to it) represented local public health providers, general practitioners, mental health services, third-sector organisations, faith groups, private providers (e.g. of exercise programmes), the local council and – most importantly for this chapter – citizens (older people, young mothers, mental health service users and so on). There was much debate –about what was happening locally (What exactly *was* the problem we were trying to solve – and how should we measure it?), about the research evidence (Did randomised trials exist – and should we expect them to exist – on every aspect of the problem?) and most of all about what we should *do*. A powerful piece of evidence was a video made by a small voluntary-sector organisation in which older people described how hard it was to access health services and the impact this had on their health and well-being.

One issue that interested our health inequalities commission was the question of 'social prescribing' – an umbrella term for advising people with complex health and/or social needs to take up a non-medical service (e.g. linking with a 'good neighbours' scheme or joining a weight-watchers club). Social prescribing was not something I knew much about, and my own reading of the academic literature was that the evidence base on its efficacy was limited [30]. But there was already money on the table locally to 'pilot' some form of social prescribing with a view to redressing health inequalities. Gradually, the various stakeholders reached broad agreement on what we meant by the term, what was already happening locally and what we would like to do as a new piece of applied research.

The social prescribing study we planned (and which is now ongoing) is not the one that I would have done if given a blank canvas, the existing research evidence and an unconstrained budget. Rather, it is a compromise between my own views on what the academic knowledge gap was, what others around the table wanted to study, what the patient groups had said were their priorities and – very significantly – what we were allowed to spend the money on. I doubt if the findings from this humble study will end up getting published in the *Lancet*. But – and here is where Mode 2 research sometimes leapfrogs over Mode 1 – they will have immediate salience and importance to the local stakeholders who designed the study. If we find that something 'works' and is affordable, that something will almost certainly move seamlessly into practice.

This example (which is a work in progress) illustrates a key characteristic of co-designed (Mode 2) research: a wide range of perspectives and practical approaches – including but not limited to clever theory and specialist scientific techniques – are mobilised and managed, often for a limited period only, to address a particular set of problems. Planning, execution, dissemination and implementation of research are not separate and linear phases, but interwoven. The relationship between scientists and research users (policymakers, citizens and so on) is one of co-production rather than producer–consumer or contractor–commissioner.

If you want to read more about co-created research, I have co-authored reviews of the literature on co-creation in general [31] and of community-based participatory research in particular [20].

6.5 Communicating research: whose literacy is the problem?

Research is a complex business; many people do not understand it. The traditional (now discredited) view is that scientists are very clever, whilst 'lay' people are less clever and may lack the understanding or vocabulary to grasp what scientists do. A more contemporary view is that if a researcher cannot explain what they have done (or plan to do) to a randomly selected individual of average intelligence, they probably don't fully understand it themselves either. Sometimes, it's not quite that simple. I will never get my head round string theory, whoever explains it.

One thing is not in doubt: on a scale of outstanding to terrible, many researchers are close to terrible at communicating the rationale for their research (e.g. Why this study? Why now? Why on these participants?), its design (e.g. What is a randomised trial and why are we using this approach?), key aspects of the method (e.g. Why do the participants have to have a blood test every month?), its main findings (e.g. Did the drug work? If so, in what ways and with what caveats?) and its implications (How, if at all, should practice change?) to people outside their ivory-tower world.

How do I know that? For one thing, I once sat on a committee that assessed 'lay summaries' of research as part of a wider remit. I could not understand most of them myself, and researchers' rather patronising efforts to use 'lay language' often made my toes curl. The things researchers painstakingly explained in short sentences were not actually the bits I had trouble understanding. I wanted to know why the particular piece of research being described *mattered*. What had been done by previous researchers to make *this* study the obvious next step? These were things that most researchers considered self-evident, so did not explain.

There has not been much research on lay summaries of either planned or published research, but the few available studies confirm that many such summaries are opaque to the lay reader (and by 'lay' I mean anyone outside the immediate field). A systematic review of recruitment of patients into clinical trials, for example, found widespread misunderstanding of terms such as 'randomisation', 'placebo', 'benefit' and 'risk' [32]. Only 3 of 27 studies included in that review had undertaken any assessment of the readability of the patient information sheet or consent form. Whilst one study has shown that people volunteering for research make their decisions intuitively and based largely on trust (in the researchers and in the organisation where the research is undertaken) [33], few researchers would use that finding to justify pulling the wool over patients' eyes.

A small study of the comprehensibility of Cochrane review lay summaries recruited university staff as their 'lay' readers; exactly a third understood the abstract; just over half understood the 'lay summary'; and 78% understood an audio podcast made by the authors of the study [34]. In another study, student midwives understood around 60% of both abstracts and lay summaries of Cochrane reviews [35]. The Cochrane Collaboration is leading the field in a major initiative to improve the writing of what they refer to as 'plain language summaries'. You can access the Cochrane Plain Language Summaries website here: http://community.cochrane.org/style-manual/cochrane-review-specific/plain-language-summaries the Norwegian Cochrane centre has produced a downloadable guide to writing such summaries [36].

It is worth asking patients and lay people to help you write summaries. We know that involving lay people in the development of patient information materials makes those materials more relevant, readable and understandable [37]. When patients with a condition explain things to other patients with the same condition, they often start from exactly where that individual is coming from – and that can be a firm foundation for generating understanding, even if some of the scientific small print gets omitted or distorted. Ahmed Rashid and colleagues have recently published a review of the literature on how patient and lay involvement can improve the readability (and patient relevance) of that most turgid of literary genres – the clinical guideline [38].

There is another aspect of research communication that I have barely touched on in this book, and that is the wider issue of public engagement by scientists. INVOLVE defines engagement as the process by which information and knowledge about research is provided and disseminated [1]. People do not just need to know what is happening in *this particular* research study; they need to understand research in general (Why, for example, do some of us think randomised controlled trials are such a good thing?) or they will never be able to give informed consent to their own participation or have meaningful input into the prioritisation of research topics.

Examples of engagement are:

- science festivals open to the public with debates and discussions on research;
- open days at research centres to which members of the public are invited to find out about research;
- raising awareness of research through media such as television, newspapers and social media;
- dissemination to research participants, colleagues or members of the public on the findings of a study.

When I was researching this book, I discovered a diverse and hotly contested literature on how (and how not) to undertake public engagement activities like these. Whilst it is an interesting and important topic, I fear it needs a book all of its own, so I have not done a deep dive into that literature here. Interested readers might like to start with a recent introductory essay by Jack Stilgoe and Simon Lock [39].

6.6 Ten tips for improving citizen involvement in research

1. Persuade yourself that citizen involvement matters
Too many researchers see 'PPI' as a tick in a box. Look up the papers referenced in Section 6.1 on the evidence base showing that involving lay partners in research is our ethical duty *and* will probably improve the quality, efficiency and ultimate impact of our work. The extent to which you care about this will determine how well you deliver on it.

2. Use the right terminology
Use Table 6.1 to distinguish between 'patients', 'citizens', 'service users' and so on. Choose the word that best matches what you're trying to do, with whom and why. Above all, expunge the word 'subject' from your vocabulary unless you have a very specific and legitimate reason to be using it.

3. Understand what excellent looks like
Look at the different taxonomies of lay involvement in Section 6.2. Are you, for example, seeking to involve lay people in your research nominally (i.e. just to say you have done it), instrumentally (to achieve particular goals and steps in your research study), representatively (in addition to delivering on your project, to build capacity for research involvement amongst lay people

and communities) or transformatively (to enable particular groups to *set* the research agenda and thereby influence their own destiny)? Not all research needs to be user-led and transformative, but that is (arguably) where the bar for excellence sits

4. Prioritise research questions that patients themselves pose

See Section 6.3 for examples of how patients can suggest game-changers to the research agenda. If you do not know about the JLA and the HTA programme's research suggestions portal, get surfing and check out their websites.

5. Conduct research with, not on, patients

This chapter should have persuaded you that involvement of patients and citizens can occur at all stages of the research journey, including in setting research priorities, study design, choice of outcome measures, recruitment, study implementation, interpretation of findings and dissemination. A diverse and questioning steering group may help recruit more diverse and representative samples and head off potential ethical problems before they occur. Involving groups rather than individuals (see Figure 6.1) will strengthen the patient/lay voice.

6. Go further: co-create research

Mode 2 research (Section 6.4) is radical stuff for most doctors, but co-created research with citizens has been happening for decades in other fields. If your research questions (or, better, the research questions your patients and community groups are coming up with) are about how to improve things for a local underserved group, Mode 2 might be just the ticket.

7. Learn to write (and speak) in plain English

Most researchers open their mouths and talk jargon, and they do even worse when putting pen to paper (see Section 6.5). Look back at the tips in Section 2.5 on shortening, sharpening, tailoring, narrativising and visualising your message. Above all, keep practising – like any writing genre, lay summary-writing improves the more you do it.

8. Involve patients, citizens and the lay media in disseminating research findings

As I briefly mentioned in Section 6.5, patients and citizens are often better than we scientists and clinicians at explaining things to other patients. That is not necessarily the case – but if you can find yourself a lay partner who can weave the words, your lay summaries will reach the parts other lay summaries manifestly fail to.

9. Get out more

You are not going to get better at communicating your research if you sit in your office all day. Accept that invitation to give a talk to a school (or community group or patient group), speak in a debate, go on the radio or record a podcast of your new paper. Don't be shy: practice makes perfect.

10. Invite the public in

If you do research and have not yet had a 'research day' to which you invite the public, give it a go. It will be hard work – and you will learn a lot about the logistics of such events – but I predict you will also come away with a stronger sense of *why* (and for *whom*) you are doing research, and also what your target audience really cares about. This will (or should) inform your plans for your next study.

References

1. INVOLVE (2012). What Is Public Involvement in Research? Available from: http://www.invo.org.uk/find-out-more/what-is-pub (last accessed 14 January 2017).
2. Edelman, N., & Barron, D. (2015). Evaluation of public involvement in research: time for a major re-think? *Journal of Health Services Research & Policy*, **21**(3), 209–211.
3. Oliver, S.R., Rees, R.W., Clarke-Jones, L., Milne, R., Oakley, A.R., Gabbay, J., et al. (2008). A multidimensional conceptual framework for analysing public involvement in health services research. *Health Expectations*, **11**(1), 72–84.
4. Boote, J., Telford, R., & Cooper, C. (2002). Consumer involvement in health research: a review and research agenda. *Health Policy*, **61**(2), 213–236.
5. Caron-Flinterman, J.F., Broerse, J.E., & Bunders, J.F. (2005). The experiential knowledge of patients: a new resource for biomedical research? *Social Science & Medicine*, **60**(11), 2575–2584.
6. Chalmers, I., Bracken, M.B., Djulbegovic, B., Garattini, S., Grant, J., Gülmezoglu, A.M., et al. (2014). How to increase value and reduce waste when research priorities are set. *Lancet*, **383**(9912), 156–165.
7. Entwistle, V., Calnan, M., & Dieppe, P. (2008). Consumer involvement in setting the health services research agenda: persistent questions of value. *Journal of Health Services Research & Policy*, **13**(Suppl. 3), 76–81.
8. Staley, K. (2009). *Exploring Impact: Public Involvement in NHS, Public Health and Social Care Research*. National Institute for Health Research.
9. Staley, K., & Doherty, C. (2016). It's not evidence, it's insight: bringing patients' perspectives into health technology appraisal at NICE. *Research Involvement and Engagement*, **2**(1), 1.
10. Barnes, M., Harrison, S., Mort, M., & Shardlow, P. (1999). *Unequal Partners: User Groups and Community Care*. Bristol, The Policy Press.
11. Hogg, C., & Williamson, C. (2001). Whose interests do lay people represent? Towards an understanding of the role of lay people as members of committees. *Health Expectations*, **4**(1), 2–9.

Chapter 6

12. Popay, J., & Collins, M. (2014). *Public Involvement Impact Assessment Framework.* Available from: http://piiaf.org.uk/# (last accessed 4 March 2017).
13. Kristjansson, E.A., Robinson, V., Petticrew, M., MacDonald, B., Krasevec, J., Janzen, L., et al. (2007). School feeding for improving the physical and psychosocial health of disadvantaged elementary school children. *Cochrane Database of Systematic Reviews*, 1:CD004676.
14. Gradinger, F., Britten, N., Wyatt, K., Froggatt, K., Gibson, A., Jacoby, A., et al. (2015). Values associated with public involvement in health and social care research: a narrative review. *Health Expectations*, 18(5), 661–675.
15. Arnstein, S.R. (1969). A ladder of citizen participation. *Journal of the American Institute of Planners*, 35(4), 216–224.
16. Tritter, J.Q., & McCallum, A. (2006). The snakes and ladders of user involvement: moving beyond Arnstein. *Health Policy*, 76(2), 156–168.
17. Cornwall, A. (2008). Unpacking 'participation': models, meanings and practices. *Community Development Journal*, 43(3), 269–283.
18. White, S.C. (1996). Depoliticising development: the uses and abuses of participation. *Development in Practice*, 6(1), 6–15.
19. Research Design Service (2014). Public Involvement. Available from: http://www.rds.nihr.ac.uk/public-involvement/(last accessed 14 January 2017).
20. Jagosh, J., Macaulay, A.C., Pluye, P., Salsberg, J., Bush, P.L., Henderson, J., et al. (2012). Uncovering the benefits of participatory research: implications of a realist review for health research and practice. *The Milbank Quarterly*, 90(2), 311–346.
21. Vieira, H.P., Leite, I.A., Sampaio, T.M.A., de Paula, J.d.A., do Nascimento Andrade, A., de Abreu, L.C., et al. (2013). Bisphosphonates adherence for treatment of osteoporosis. *International Archives of Medicine*, 6(1), 1.
22. Li, M., Zhang, Z.L., Liao, E.Y., Chen, D.C., Liu, J., Tao, T.Z., et al. Effect of low-dose alendronate treatment on bone mineral density and bone turnover markers in Chinese postmenopausal women with osteopenia and osteoporosis. *Menopause (New York, NY)*, 20(1), 72–78.
23. Deane, K.H., Flaherty, H., Daley, D.J., Pascoe, R., Penhale, B., Clarke, C.E., et al. (2014). Priority setting partnership to identify the top 10 research priorities for the management of Parkinson's disease. *BMJ Open*, 4(12):e006434.
24. Snow, R., Crocker, J., & Crowe, S. (2015). Missed opportunities for impact in patient and carer involvement: a mixed methods case study of research priority setting. *Research Involvement and Engagement*, 1(1), 1.
25. Piil, K., & Jarden, M. (2016). Patient Involvement in Research Priorities (PIRE): a study protocol. *BMJ Open*, 6(5), e010615.
26. Dawson, J., Doll, H., Fitzpatrick, R., Jenkinson, C., & Carr, A.J. (2010). The routine use of patient reported outcome measures in healthcare settings. *BMJ*, 340, c186.
27. Shippee, N.D., Domecq Garces, J.P., Prutsky Lopez, G.J., Wang, Z., Elraiyah, T.A., Nabhan, M., et al. (2015). Patient and service user engagement in research: a systematic review and synthesized framework. *Health Expectations*, 18(5), 1151–1166.
28. Gibbons, M., Limoges, C., Nowotny, H., Schwartzman, S., Scott, P., & Trow, M. (1994). *The New Production of Knowledge: The Dynamics of Science and Research in Contemporary Societies.* London, Sage.

29. Nowotny, H., Scott, P., & Gibbons, M. (2003). Mode 2 revisited: the new production of knowledge. *Minerva*, **41**(3), 179–194.

30. Husk, K., Blockley, K., Lovell, R., Bethel, A., Bloomfield, D., Warber, S., et al. (2016). What approaches to social prescribing work, for whom, and in what circumstances? A protocol for a realist review. *Systematic Reviews*, **5**(1), 1.

31. Greenhalgh, T., Jackson, C., Shaw, S., & Janaiman, T. (2016). Achieving research impact through co-creation in community-based health services: literature review and case study. *The Milbank Quarterly*, **94**(2), 392–429.

32. Montalvo, W., & Larson, E. (2014). Participant comprehension of research for which they volunteer: a systematic review. *Journal of Nursing Scholarship*, **46**(6), 423–431.

33. Dixon-Woods, M., Ashcroft, R.E., Jackson, C.J., Tobin, M.D., Kivits, J., Burton, P.R., & Samani, N.J. (2007). Beyond 'misunderstanding': written information and decisions about taking part in a genetic epidemiology study. *Social Science & Medicine*, **65**(11), 2212–2222.

34. Maguire, L.K., & Clarke, M. (2014). How much do you need: a randomised experiment of whether readers can understand the key messages from summaries of Cochrane Reviews without reading the full review. *Journal of the Royal Society of Medicine*, **107**(11), 444–449.

35. Alderdice, F., McNeill, J., Lasserson, T., Beller, E., Carroll, M., Hundley, V., et al. (2016). Do Cochrane summaries help student midwives understand the findings of Cochrane systematic reviews: the BRIEF randomised trial. *Systematic Reviews*, **5**(1), 1.

36. Glenton, C. (2016). How to Write a Lay Summary of a Cochrane Intervention Review. Available from: http://www.cochrane.no/sites/cochrane.no/files/public/uploads/How%20to%20write%20a%20Cochrane%20PLS%209th%20June%202016.pdf (last accessed 14 January 2017).

37. Nilsen, E.S., Myrhaug, H.T., Johansen, M., Oliver, S., & Oxman, A.D. (2006). Methods of consumer involvement in developing healthcare policy and research, clinical practice guidelines and patient information material. *Cochrane Database of Systematic Reviews*, **3**:CD004563.

38. Rashid, A., Thomas, V., Price, T., & Leng, G. (2017). Patient and public involvement in the development of healthcare guidance and quality indicators. *Under review*.

39. Stilgoe, J., Lock, S.J., & Wilsdon, J. (2014). Why should we promote public engagement with science? *Public Understanding of Science*, **23**(1), 4–15.

Chapter 6

Chapter 7 **Patients**

7.1 Is the EBHC movement biased against patients?

Not long ago, along with some co-authors, I wrote a paper entitled 'Six "Biases" against Patients and Carers in Evidence-Based Medicine' [1]. What on earth did we mean by suggesting that evidence-based medicine (EBM) was 'biased'? Surely evidence-based anything is the science of trying to *avoid* bias? Let me explain.

Take the standard sequence of how research happens. First, researchers (with or without the input from patients and citizens that I covered in Chapter 6) decide which outcomes will count. When looking at diabetes prevention programmes, for example, are we interested in weight gain, haemoglobin A1c (HbA1c) levels or the development of full-blown type 2 diabetes? Then, an empirical study (or perhaps a systematic review) is done to find out how to best achieve those outcomes. The results of such studies are written up for publication. Sometime later, a clinician interprets and (hopefully) shares the findings with their patient in the clinical encounter.

But as we pointed out in the 'Six Biases' paper, the patient in this scenario begins from a different place. Even when patients are 'informed', 'empowered' and 'health-literate' (and especially when they are not), they rarely inhabit a world of controlled experiments, objective measurement of predefined outcomes, average results or generalisable truths. Rather, they live in the messy, idiosyncratic and unpredictable world of a particular person in a particular family context (or, for some, in a context of social isolation and/or abandonment by family). Notwithstanding this, patients may seek out medical information and self-monitor their own tests and treatments, with or without the knowledge or support of their clinician.

After seeing the doctor, nurse, pharmacist or other healthcare professional (and perhaps taking part in a more or less shared decision about what to do), the patient goes away and re-enters what has been termed the 'lifeworld' – a world populated by people rather than biomedical variables, where what

How to Implement Evidence-Based Healthcare, First Edition. Trisha Greenhalgh.
© 2018 John Wiley & Sons Ltd. Published 2018 by John Wiley & Sons Ltd.

matters are particularities, not mean values or generalisable truths. In this unique world, different things will inevitably be at stake from the ones selected as primary or secondary outcome measures in a research study.

As the excellent website www.healthtalk.org illustrates through video narratives from real patients, the illness *as lived* differs considerably from the disease or risk state in the evidence-based guideline. With the help of family, friends and peers, the patient (or, more accurately, *person*, since they are a patient only when experiencing care in the healthcare system) will try to align the evidence-based model of disease with the actual experience of illness or (assigned) risk. And as a Canadian team has recently shown, it may be the *unintended* consequences of interventions that most help and hinder people living with illness [2].

Six features of evidence-based healthcare (EBHC) – which we referred to in our paper, figuratively, as 'biases' – may inadvertently devalue this broader patient and carer agenda [1]:

Bias 1. Lack of patient input to the research process: As indicated in the previous chapter, it is still rare for citizens to have a major say in the design and execution of clinical research studies. As a result, endpoints of trials may reflect what researchers find easy to measure rather than what matters most to patients. Side effects of treatments (e.g. hypoglycaemia in intensive insulin therapy) may be treated lightly because researchers simply do not understand how troubling they are, having never experienced them themselves.

Bias 2. The low status given to experience ('anecdote') in the hierarchy of evidence: Anecdote (a story about one individual) is rightly placed at the bottom of the hierarchy of evidence when assessing what kinds of research are generalisable to a different patient. The story of your uncle who smoked 40 a day till he died at 98 is *not* proof that cigarette smoking is a safe habit. But an anecdote (i.e. honest account) of what is happening in *this* patient is hugely important. It is what I like to call 'personally significant evidence' for decision-making in relation to that particular patient.

Bias 3. An expectation that 'tools' are the answer: There is a tendency amongst some members of the EBHC community to conflate patient-centred care with the use of shared decision-making tools – which sometimes depict the key decisions in very biomedical terms. I am not at all opposed to such tools (see Section 7.2, where I sing their praises), but let us not forget that they may have been designed around the doctor's or the researcher's agenda, not the patient's.

Bias 4. Underemphasis on power: The EBHC community gives only limited attention to power imbalances that suppress the patient's voice. Hands up those whose elderly relative will not say anything which he or she thinks might upset or challenge the doctor, for example. Unless we acknowledge that patients may not say what they really think because most of the power in the consultation lies with the clinician, we will never get true sharing of information or decisions.

Bias 5. **Overemphasis on what goes on in the clinical encounter:** EBHC has tended to overemphasise decisions that happen in the clinical encounter whilst overlooking such things as the ongoing work of self-management, the importance of the patient's wider social networks (including friends, neighbours and online self-help groups) and the wider input of healthcare team members, including pharmacists, healthcare assistants and receptionists.

Bias 6. **Overlooking the hidden denominator:** EBHC's primary focus is on people who seek and obtain care, rather than on people who do not seek or cannot access care – for example, because they live on the margins of society. The people with the worst outcome for just about any disease are those who lack full citizenship status (e.g. refugees, asylum seekers and illegal immigrants). These individuals may not be registered in the healthcare systems that provide the cohorts for observational studies or the sampling frame for randomised trials.

If you are interested in exploring these 'biases' in more detail, the paper is freely available online [1]. The rest of this chapter considers how the clinical encounter and self-care by people living with illness outside the clinical encounter might better incorporate the best research evidence.

7.2 Implementing evidence with patients in the clinical encounter

We all know we are supposed to have evidence-informed, non-paternalistic conversations with patients about the options for investigating and managing the conditions that concern them (and also, perhaps, about the conditions and risk states that may or may not concern them). But how do we make this ideal a reality?

There has been a generation of research into shared decision-making tools that present evidence on the benefits, potential side effects and costs of different management options. Adrian Edwards and Glyn Elwyn provide numerous examples in their book, *Shared Decision-Making in Health Care* [3]. Let me give you one of my own. In Section 6.2, I shared a recent dilemma from my own experience as a patient: Should I keep taking alendronate to protect me from the consequences of low bone density (which runs in my family)? On the plus side, this drug has been shown to be effective in reducing bone loss; on the minus side, it was giving me minor but annoying side effects. As I contemplated whether to keep taking the drug or not, I was introduced to a decision aid developed by Victor Montori and his team at the Mayo Clinic Shared Decision-Making Resource Center in the United States (http://shareddecisions.mayoclinic.org). From the menu, I selected 'osteoporosis' (a condition that I don't yet have, but if I don't look after myself I'll end up with it) and entered some data, including my age, gender, fracture history and femoral neck bone density.

Figure 7.1 shows the report I generated by putting these details into the online tool. Using simple pictograms and colour-coding, the decision tool depicted my absolute risk of developing a hip fracture over the next 10 years as 10% if I do not take my medication – and 6% if I do. It also allowed me to get a visual estimate of *relative* risk reduction: if I take the drug, the risk goes down from 10 per hundred to only 6 per hundred – a reduction of 40%. Given that I am still spending a lot of time on my racing bike, I have decided to tolerate the side effects as a worthwhile trade-off for that benefit. Note that I worked all this out at home on my own (using my background medical and epidemiological knowledge to help interpret the diagrams), but Mayo Clinic

Chapter 7

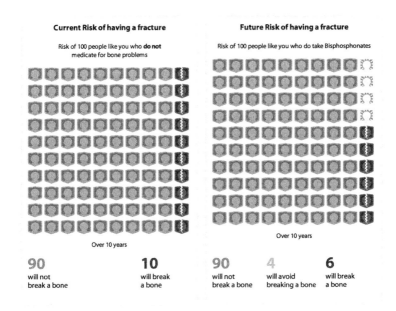

Figure 7.1 Example of a patient decision aid (on osteoporosis). *Source:* Generated using online tool at http://shareddecisions.mayoclinic.org.

tools are designed to be used within the clinical consultation, with both patient and clinician looking at the screen together.

I timed how long it took me to use the decision aid shown in Figure 7.1: less than 5 minutes, including time spent familiarising myself with the website and digging out the result of my last bone density scan. If I had had to look up the research evidence myself, my search would have taken many hours. I trust the decision aid because I know that Victor Montori's team is made up of world leaders in EBHC. But not all decision aids have such excellent provenance – and 'clear' diagrams are no use unless the evidence on which they are based is robust and up to date. The field has developed to the extent that there is now an agreed set of international standards for patient decision tools [4].

A systematic review led by Glyn Elwyn summarises evidence on the efficacy of patient decision tools (there is a great deal of evidence that they increase patients' knowledge, understanding and confidence) and on the implementation of such tools in the real world (in general, clinicians do not use them) [5]. The three main reasons that clinicians give for this mismatch are lack of time, lack of clinical applicability (the clinician believes that the patient in front of them differs significantly from the population sample on which the research was done) and the microdynamics of the consultation (which rarely unfolds as an exercise in probabilistic decision science) [6].

In Section 7.1, I introduced the term 'personally significant evidence'. We are all unique individuals, with both physiological and psychological idiosyncrasies. Almost none of us gets ill or responds to treatment in the same way as the Mr or Ms Average represented in clinical guidelines, however evidence-based those guidelines are. But – and this is an important principle that is given too little emphasis in EBHC – even when we are 'outliers' compared to the group average, we are often consistent with our own individual pattern.

Here is an example. Non-steroidal anti-inflammatory drugs (NSAIDs) often cause gastrointestinal side effects, especially when taken on an empty stomach – but they do not cause them in me. I could consume them like Smarties (although please be assured I don't). What is more, they work well for me at controlling all sorts of aches and pains. I have a friend for whom the opposite is true: she gets dreadful bellyache on NSAIDs and they do not control her pain very well. The *best* evidence about the benefits and side effects of NSAIDs *for each of us* is our own individual experience, not the published result of a randomised trial on some other group of people. Clinicians so often dismiss personal stories out of hand because they have been inoculated with the word 'anecdote' and have made conceptual antibodies against the term. Yet personally significant evidence from the patient should often, if not always, trump statistically significant evidence from a distant research study.

I want to bring in values. Different people are concerned about different aspects of a set of decision options. Some women with early breast cancer, for example, cannot wait to have a mastectomy because they want to feel fully shot of the cancer; others are desperately concerned about the wholeness of their body and want to preserve their breast (or, if that is not possible, their nipple) at all costs. The trade-offs are different for each individual because people value things differently. Figure 7.2 shows an option grid, developed by Glyn Elwyn's team, which is designed to be printed off and given to the patient to take home whilst they think about their choices. The same tool was converted to a simple picture format after a co-design process with lay people whose health literacy was low [7].

There is a growing evidence base showing that patient decision tools work only when used flexibly to *support conversations* rather than *dictate practice* [8]. Contrary to the assumptions of many in the EBHC community, the clinical

Breast cancer: surgical options

Use this **Option Grid**™ decision aid to help you and your healthcare professional talk about how best to treat breast cancer.

Frequently Asked Questions ↓	Lumpectomy with radiotherapy	Mastectomy
What is removed?	The cancer lump is removed, with some surrounding tissue.	The whole breast is removed.
Which surgery is best for long-term survival?	Survival rates are the same for both options.	Survival rates are the same for both options.
What are the chances of cancer coming back in the breast?	Breast cancer will come back in the breast in about 10 in every 100 women (10%) in the 10 years after a lumpectomy. Recent improvements in treatment may have reduced this risk.	Breast cancer will come back in the area of the scar in about 5 in every 100 women (5%) in the 10 years after a mastectomy. Recent improvements in treatment may have reduced this risk.
Will I need more than one operation on the breast?	Possibly, if there are still cancer cells in the breast after the lumpectomy. This can occur in up to 20 in every 100 (20%) women.	No, unless you choose breast reconstruction
How long will it take to recover?	Most women are home within 24 hours of surgery.	Most women are home within 48 hours after surgery.
Will I need radiotherapy?	Yes, for up to six weeks after surgery	Radiotherapy is not usually given after mastectomy.
Will I need to have my lymph glands removed?	Some or all of the lymph glands in the armpit are usually removed.	Some or all of the lymph glands in the armpit are usually removed.
Will I need chemotherapy?	You may be offered chemotherapy, but this does not depend on the operation you choose.	You may be offered chemotherapy, but this does not depend on the operation you choose.
Will I lose my hair?	Hair loss is common after chemotherapy.	Hair loss is common after chemotherapy.

*Under Revision: March 2016

Figure 7.2 Example of an option grid (on surgical options for early breast cancer). *Source:* http://optiongrid.org/option-grids/grid-landing/9.

encounter is not (wholly) an exercise in rational decision science. We make many of our healthcare choices for non-rational reasons – for example, because we think a particular option would fit in with family plans, align with cultural expectations of good parenting or honour the memory of an ancestor [9]. Unless these reasons are recognised as primary drivers of human behaviour, clinician and patient will be at cross-purposes.

Communication is only partly about sharing information and agreeing a management plan; it also involves talk and gestures aimed at establishing and strengthening a therapeutic relationship [10]. The therapeutic relationship is central, not marginal, to evidence-based practice. The stronger it is, the greater the chance that there will be a mutually agreed management plan, the more comfortable the patient will be carrying out their part in the plan and the more satisfied both parties will be [11].

There is strong and consistent evidence that the success of the evidence-based consultation depends as much on its humanistic elements as on what information is shared and how. It is nearly 30 years since family medicine introduced the 'patient centred clinical method' [12,13], summarised in a recent review as:

> *the adoption of a biopsychosocial [incorporating EBHC, psychology and attention to social context] perspective by providers; the sharing of decisions and responsibilities between patients and providers; the strengthening of practitioners' compassion, sensitivity to patients' distress and commitment to respond to patients with empathy in an effort to alleviate suffering.* [14]

As Miles and Mezzich have observed, the EBHC movement (oriented to objective, scientific and often mathematical management of disease and risk) and the movement for patient-centred care ('the … imperative to care, comfort and console as well as to ameliorate, attenuate and cure') have emerged in parallel rather than in dialogue with one another [15]. The time is well overdue for these two important streams of scholarship in clinical method to explore their differences and establish common ground.

A final factor to consider in relation to the clinical encounter is power. As my colleagues and I argue in the 'Six biases' paper, healthcare interactions are characterised by socially prescribed roles and by imbalances of power and status that profoundly affect how each party behaves [1]. Even in situations where patients know more than the doctor treating them about their particular condition, the power dynamic is such that patients may say nothing, or say what they hope the doctor wants to hear. When patients do speak freely, the doctor's evidence tends to trump the patient's evidence (e.g. in arguments about whether a symptom is cause by a drug side effect).

More recently, it has been pointed out that many clinical decisions these days get made outside the clinician–patient encounter. For example, these days cancer tends to be managed by multidisciplinary teams (MDTs). It is often in the MDT meeting (behind closed doors) that the uncertainties about a case are discussed and a provisional decision is made; one clinician then takes on the task of conveying this decision to the patient [16]. It would be a rare and brave patient who would be prepared to challenge this 'done deal', especially when made vulnerable by a new diagnosis of cancer.

I firmly believe that EBHC needs to pay more nuanced attention to power dynamics. In the 'Six biases' paper, we summarise the (currently, fairly sparse) evidence base for measures that can help redress the impact of such power imbalances – such as allocating more time to the consultation, using advocates and mediators, encouraging patients to bring lists of concerns, explicitly recognising and addressing the differing needs of disadvantaged groups and visiting vulnerable patients in their homes [1].

I would like to see more research, especially qualitative studies informed by the social sciences, on how to align evidence-based decision support with true power-sharing in clinical care. Glyn Elwyn, Sietse Wieringa and I recently wrote a (somewhat speculative) paper on what the clinical encounter might look like in what we call the 'post-guidelines era' – a time in the (hopefully) not-too-distant future when the democratic use of evidence-based decision aids has become part of business as usual [17].

7.3 Self-management and how to support it

Sharing decisions in the clinical encounter is important, but this framing assumes that the key interactions happen between a patient and a clinician around a medical decision tree. In fact, most illness management – including most decision-making about care – happens at home, by a person living with illness, with input from their family and carer(s), when the clinician is not present. Such activities have come to be known as 'self-management'.

The research literature on self-management and how best to support it can be divided more or less cleanly into two camps (although some researchers, notably Professor Anne Rogers, have managed to keep a foot in both). There is research that begins with the clinician's view of what is needed and is built around a biomedical main course, often with a side salad of psychological theory [18]. And there is a quite different research tradition that begins with the patient in his or her lifeworld and sits more comfortably in the social sciences and humanities, using narrative and naturalistic research methods (such as ethnography) [19].

You could say that biomedical research looks at self-management of *disease* whereas the lifeworld model is more interested in self-management of *illness* (illness being what you have when you are on your way to see the doctor; disease being what you have on your way home). Traditional EBHC (the findings from clinical trials, observational studies and diagnostic test validation) is important to both, but it aligns more closely with the former. Depending on your mental model of self-management, the evidence-based solutions you find will be very different.

I recently played a small role in a team that reviewed the literature on self-management in chronic disease [18]. It was a massive task, since the topic has been extensively researched. We noted that self-management has been defined by the UK Department of Health in its Expert Patient Programme (from what I would call a predominantly biomedical perspective that pays passing acknowledgement to the lifeworld) as 'developing the confidence and motivation of patients to use their own skills and knowledge to take effective control over life with a chronic illness'; it emphasises that this is 'not simply about educating or instructing patients about their condition' [20].

Drawing on earlier work by others, our review team considered three aspects of self-management: medical management (making decisions, complying with medication, doing one's physiotherapy exercises and so on), role management (getting used to the restrictions on lifestyle associated with a chronic condition and negotiating such things as time off work) and emotional management (dealing with one's own and others' emotional reactions) [18]. Professor Kate Lorig, a nurse by background who led the field in randomised trials of self-management support, identified five core sets of skills to address these three kinds of self-management:

1. problem-solving;
2. decision-making;
3. appropriate resource utilisation;
4. forming a partnership with a health-care provider;
5. taking necessary actions [21].

The assumptions behind much of Lorig's work – which informed and underpinned the UK Expert Patient Programme of self-management education and set a pattern that most subsequent research teams have followed – is that someone with a chronic condition will be able to effectively self-manage only when he or she has acquired a particular set of skills; that these skills can be acquired through a structured programme of self-management education (led either by professionals or by fellow patients who have been trained in the method); and that the mechanism by which self-management *education* leads to self-management *behaviours* is through a gain in *self-efficacy* (which I defined and discussed in Section 3.2).

Lorig and others have shown in numerous well-designed randomised controlled trials and across numerous different chronic diseases that patients who attend this kind of self-management training usually gain in self-efficacy, demonstrate improved skill at a predefined set of tasks and (sometimes) achieve improvements in biomarkers such as blood pressure or HbA1c [18]. Despite this evidence, I still worry that this whole field of research is overly behaviourist in its focus and is missing the essence of what it *really* means to suffer from, live with and manage an incurable, serious, lifelong illness.

Take a systematic review of group-based self-management education for diabetes by Steinsbekk et al. [22], for example. I quote from the abstract (from which I have removed the numerical values for ease of reading):

> For the main clinical outcomes, HbA1c was significantly reduced at 6 months, 12 months and 2 years and fasting blood glucose levels were also significantly reduced at 12 months but not at 6 months. For the main lifestyle outcomes, diabetes knowledge was improved significantly at 6 months, 12 months and 2 years and self-management skills also improved significantly at 6 months. For the main psychosocial outcomes, there were significant improvement[s] for empowerment/self-efficacy after 6 months. For quality of life no conclusion could be drawn due to high heterogeneity. (p. 213)

I think the reason why these findings do not excite me is that I am firmly in the 'lifeworld' camp for self-management research. I am sure self-efficacy and performance of self-management tasks, as defined by researchers, are important. But I also know that there are dozens of other things that matter to people – and that these will be different for different individuals and hence impossible to abstract into a single, easily measurable variable [23]. I am also cynical that a key goal in most self-management support studies is to reduce care utilisation [24] – as if success equates with how far biomedical care tasks and their associated costs can be shifted from the healthcare system to the patient. Social scientists have shown that health service utilisation by self-managing patients is a lot more complex than that [25].

Most importantly, I do not wholeheartedly buy into the 'deficit' and 'behaviour change' model on which expert patient research is predicated (the patient is depicted as deficient in an abstracted set of problem-solving skills, decision-making skills, self-efficacy and so on, and it is presumed that he or she will be better off when and to the extent that these deficits come to be redressed through structured education). The deficit model ignores evidence that almost all patients know more than their clinician about their illnesses – if by 'knowledge' we mean the subjective, embodied knowledge of how the illness actually affects them and how they respond to particular treatments [26].

Indeed, as a study of type 1 diabetes patients showed, some patients really do have more *medical* knowledge than their doctors [27]. After all, if your life depended on being up to speed on a particular and somewhat obscure corner of the biomedical literature, you would probably put the work in to familiarise yourself with it. Managing a chronic illness involves work [28], which is typically done not by the patient alone but by a distributed network of family and friends (I cover such networks in Section 10.4 [29]). Surprisingly often, it is the patient and their family who need to educate the clinician about what this work entails, not the other way around.

Whilst biomedical research into self-management support has (in my view) got itself into a bit of a rut (consisting of randomised trials testing the impact of support programme X on outcome Y, typically paying much homage to self-efficacy scores and attending little if at all to how people actually live with illness), there is now some excellent 'grey literature' that extends the paradigm in a more holistic way. The Health Foundation, for example, has produced a practical guide to supporting self-management that exhorts us to follow four principles [30]:

1. Afford people dignity, compassion and respect.
2. Offer coordinated care, support or treatment (a point which acknowledges that self-management by patients needs a flexible and responsive healthcare system, not a rigid bureaucracy in which the patient is just a number or a set of test results).
3. Offer personalised care, support or treatment (by which they mean listen to the patient, take account of his or her concerns and context, and try to go at the pace and direction set by the patient and family).
4. Support people to recognise and develop their own strengths and abilities to enable them to live an independent and fulfilling life (perhaps through an 'expert patient' course – but perhaps by other means).

These are laudable principles – but they focus mainly on the small amount of time the patient spends within the healthcare system. As Elizabeth Kendall and Anne Rogers have eloquently argued, self-management programmes and policies, even when they espouse the values of holistic care, rarely go beyond the biomedical elements of the work of self-management (shared decision-making about medical tests and treatments, promoting task-oriented behaviour and the holy grail of self-efficacy) – and in choosing this focus, they thereby 'extinguish the social' (i.e. the 'lifeworld' aspects of living with chronic illness, such as how to turn down celebratory food at a family wedding or support a spouse who has not yet come to terms with the implications of your severe heart failure) [31].

To capture 'the social', we need to get out of the clinic and visit people in their natural habitat. Contrast the focus of the preceding systematic review quote with the following description from a study led by Sue Hinder from my team, who used ethnographic methods to observe (over periods of several hours) people's efforts to self-manage their diabetes at home, at school and in the workplace [32]:

> *Self-management comprised both practical and cognitive tasks (e.g. self-monitoring, menu planning, medication adjustment) and socio-emotional ones (e.g. coping with illness, managing relatives' input, negotiating access to services or resources). Self-management was hard work, and was enabled or constrained by economic, material and socio-cultural conditions within the family, workplace and community. Some people managed their diabetes skilfully and flexibly, drawing on personal capabilities, family and social networks and the healthcare system. For others, capacity to self-manage (including overcoming economic and socio-cultural constraints) was limited by co-morbidity, cognitive ability, psychological factors (e.g. under-confidence, denial) and social capital ...*
>
> *[In conclusion,] non-engagement with self-management may make sense in the context of low personal resources (e.g. health literacy, resilience) and overwhelming personal, family and social circumstances. Success of self-management as a policy solution will be affected by interacting influences at three levels: [a] at micro level by individuals' dispositions and capabilities; [b] at meso level by roles, relationships and material conditions within the family and in the workplace, school and healthcare organisation; and [c] at macro level by prevailing economic conditions, cultural norms and expectations, and the underpinning logic of the healthcare system.*

I hope you can see that when we study what people *actually* do (and why they do it) to manage their chronic condition in the real world, the biomedical framing of decision-making, self-efficacy and skills for 'self-management tasks' captures only a fraction of the overall picture. Missing are the networks of peers, friends and family and the wider context in which the work of self-management is contemplated, prioritised (or not) and accorded social meaning and moral worth.

An alternative view of self-management is that it is best conceptualised not as a set of tasks to be learnt and exhibited but as a set of *social practices* (i.e. recurrent shared activities made up of bodily actions, mental schemas, meaning-systems and tacit know-how) that are deeply embedded in particular family routines and cultural traditions [33]. I will return to social practices

Chapter 7

in Section 10.4 when I talk about the importance of 'communities of practice' in supporting self-management by patients.

This section illustrates a principle that runs through this book. I have deliberately not given you a formula for ensuring that self-management support for patients is evidence-based. Rather, I have tried to convey tensions and gaps in that evidence base, including key upstream questions about whether self-management should be conceptualised in a narrowly biomedical or more holistic way – and the implications of this question for the design of research studies.

My own view, which others may not share, is that if we are to move forward in the evidence-based support of self-management, we will need to break free of the conceptual shackles that are currently constraining the development of new ideas in this field. In particular, I would like us to move on from the view that the gold standard in this field is a randomised trial of educational intervention versus no educational intervention, with self-efficacy as the primary outcome.

7.4 Patient involvement in service improvement

Both the principles and the practicalities of patient involvement in service improvement are very similar to those on citizen involvement in research, which I covered in Chapter 6.

The United Kingdom has also pioneered the active involvement of patients and citizens in delivering clinical governance (the principle that all health services should provide the best evidence-based care). The UK Care Quality Commission (www.cqc.org.uk), for example, routinely includes lay people in the inspection teams that accredit hospitals, general practices, care homes and other National Health Service (NHS) organisations. I do not want to get distracted into an exhaustive review of the evidence on this topic. Others have done systematic reviews to show that patient-led assessments can be an effective way of driving up service quality [34], although such impact is sometimes hard to demonstrate [35].

I once co-edited a multi-author textbook on service user involvement in healthcare improvement, in which some of the chapter leads were patients and citizens and others were clinicians and/or academics [36]. We described empirical examples of patients and citizens sitting on hospital boards, collecting and analysing performance data, co-producing evidence-based information leaflets and videos for other patients, educating staff on the patient perspective and participating in experience-based co-design (see later). We found that the enthusiasm lay people had for involvement was often (although not always) high, but that institutional structures and cultures sometimes meant that they had limited influence (e.g. over how budgets were allocated or whether change was initiated).

We also highlighted an irony. Those who seek to convey to the suits on committees what it's like to be a patient will gradually acquire an institutional perspective, lose their naivety regarding the system and perhaps begin to overlook the salience of their own lifeworld perspective. There is no simple fix to this problem. As we say in the book [36]:

> All the projects struggled with the challenge of maintaining fresh engagement of service users over time and avoiding the development of a cohort of 'usual suspects' who expected to be re-invited for every new user involvement event. On the other hand, we found that with some projects, it was impractical to keep recruiting new users and that a cohort of trained and familiar individuals brought a great deal to the initiative through their accumulated experience and familiarity with the project and with one another. (p. 107)

Andrea Litva and colleagues held focus groups of lay people to explore what they perceived to be their role (and who, if anyone, they felt they were representing) in assessing clinical services [37]. Their participants held a wide range of different views and couched themselves in a range of roles (see Table 6.1). A few considered themselves to be *consumers* (asking, 'Am I getting the level of service that I expect?' – what some have called the 'choice' perspective); others viewed themselves as *advocates* ('I speak on behalf of patients with a similar condition to me, and I want to improve services for all of us' – what some have called the 'voice' perspective); others saw themselves as *citizens* ('I am committed to improving public services and/or ensuring the best use of public money'). Whichever term they used, most appeared to be motivated by a moral commitment to the public good.

This and similar studies [38,39] provide a consistent and important message: that patients and citizens want to be involved in the governance of clinical services primarily in order to convey to clinicians, managers and policymakers what the patient experience is like ('voice' rather than 'choice') and to emphasise the moral significance of the patient/lay voice to those who might be tempted to dismiss it.

As noted in the previous chapter, a central issue to consider with any lay involvement is the unequal distribution of power. The term 'patient empowerment' is ubiquitous in the literature on both research and service improvement – but it too often means 'giving patients the power to help influence things the way *we* want them to be influenced'. In such circumstances, input from lay people is carefully restricted to (for example) the narrow options that researchers, clinicians and managers have already put on the table [36]. Because of the profound power imbalance stemming from differences in status and the inherent vulnerability of being a patient (would you want to upset the person who is going to operate on your cancer if it comes back?), patients may stay quiet or assent to proposed courses of action rather than challenge them.

This was demonstrated, for example, by Carole Doherty and Charitini Stavropoulou in a systematic review of patients' willingness to become involved in patient safety initiatives [40]. Across 68 included studies, many factors (e.g. age, gender, language proficiency, illness characteristics and how busy the staff seemed to be) were identified as barriers to involvement. But perhaps the most troubling finding was that relational factors (i.e. the extent to which patients trusted their clinicians and had confidence in them) were particularly powerful disincentives. Some patients were put off by the 'hierarchical, elitist and paternalistic culture of the medical profession' (p. 260); others simply did not want to offend or challenge their doctors. The authors coined the term 'design blindness' to highlight the paradox of encouraging patients to become involved whilst ignoring the powerful social factors that militate *against* such involvement.

In short, whilst the spirit is often willing in relation to patient involvement in service improvement, the reality may lag behind, because it's hard to be democratic when power is distributed unequally. One potential way of overcoming such inherent challenges is to use a co-creation approach known as 'experience-based co-design' (EBCD) [41], which I describe in Appendix A.

7.5 Ten tips for improving evidence-based patient care

The first four tips are suggestions for improving your clinical encounters; the next two are for service improvement; and the last four are for research.

Clinical care

1. Learn more about what illness means to patients

In Section 7.1, I talked about the difference between the world of medicine and the patient's lifeworld. The illness as experienced is very different from the objective markers of disease status that form the standard currency of medical assessment. One way of learning what illness means is to read personal narratives (blogs, novels and so on) written by the ill. Another is to explore the Healthtalk website, which offers hundreds of carefully collated video clips of patient experiences, all provided with written consent (www.healthtalk.org).

2. Value and seek out personally significant evidence in the clinical encounter

In Section 7.2, I argued that 'personally significant evidence' from a particular patient in the here and now should be captured and treated as complementary to statistically significant evidence from distant research populations. When seeing patients, try to practice eliciting, recording and applying personally significant evidence.

3. Use patient decision tools when appropriate in clinical situations
Whilst we need more tools like those in Figures 7.1 and 7.2, and more adaptations of such tools for people with lower literacy levels, there are already a lot of excellent tools out there that clinicians are not using. Bookmark the Mayo Clinic Shared Decision-Making Resource Center (http://shareddecisions.mayoclinic.org) and the Option Grid website (www.optiongrid.org) for starters. Familiarise yourself with what is there and call up relevant tools when a patient is with you.

4. Improve your consultation skills more generally
In Section 7.2, I reviewed studies that showed that the use of evidence in the clinical encounter depends as much on 'soft' elements (the clinician–patient relationship, active listening and the human qualities that allow you to 'care, comfort and console') as on the 'hard' ones (use of research evidence, guidelines or patient decision tools). Reflect on your performance as a whole-person clinician as well as on how well you can do the nerdy bits. Perhaps most crucially, take power imbalance seriously – and take measures to redress it (see penultimate paragraph in Section 7.2).

Service improvement
5. Involve patients and lay people in clinical governance
The patient voice is all too often missing from initiatives to improve the quality and safety of clinical services. Yet, as noted in Section 7.4, patients and lay people add great value to boards, steering groups, evaluations, staff education programmes and so on. This is central, not marginal, to the implementation of EBHC, since the best way to promote evidence-based practice is to instil a culture of excellence – and that includes mindfulness of who we are doing this for. Remember the problem of 'design blindness' (Section 7.4) – if you put patients in a situation where they're being asked to criticise the clinicians caring for them, you may not get an honest answer. Think harder about how to protect your sources.

6. Give experience-based co-design a go
If you think you are up for using the 'emotional touch-points' from patients' stories as the trigger for improving your service, look up the EBCD approach in Appendix A and try it. I have used this approach myself to support major redesign programs – it is hard work, but fulfilling for all involved.

Research

7. Develop more evidence-based patient decision tools

Figures 7.1 and 7.2 illustrate some pretty good patient decision tools – but the available tools cover only a fraction of the decisions patients may need to make, and they have been piloted and used by only a fraction of the population (predominantly health-literate, university-educated middle-aged adults with uncomplicated textbook conditions). There is a whole generation of research to be done in order to develop, pilot and distribute tools for as many key decisions as we can find evidence for.

8. Explore how patient decision tools could be made more flexible

Notwithstanding the previous point, it is no good thinking that if we build enough patient decision tools, all decisions will be shared and become evidence-based (that did not work with guidelines, so why should it work with patient decision aids?). Unless such tools can be made more adaptable to reflect the uniqueness of each individual case, the intuitive nature of much clinical knowledge and the complex social process of team-based decision-making, they will continue to gather dust on shelves or sit unused on computers.

9. Do more qualitative research on what actually happens in the clinical encounter

As noted in Section 7.2, the clinical encounter is a complex social interaction, of which research evidence is only one component. EBHC researchers should undertake interdisciplinary, naturalistic (i.e. real-world) studies with humanities scholars and psychologists to extend and complement their current focus on evidence-based shared decision-making.

10. Do more qualitative research on what happens outside the clinical encounter

As noted in Section 7.3, living with illness is hard work – and most decisions about how to manage illness are culturally framed and happen in the context of family, school, work and extended social networks. Very few conditions have a robust evidence base regarding how people live with them in the real world – and an even less well-researched field is how people's families and others provide support (or not). Qualitative research (interviews, ethnography, close analysis of texts) is essential for building the evidence base on what actually happens and why it matters. We need to develop this evidence base – and use it to refine the care we offer and the way we design services.

References

1. Greenhalgh, T., Snow, R., Ryan, S., Rees, S., & Salisbury, H. (2015). Six 'biases' against patients and carers in evidence-based medicine. *BMC Medicine*, **13**(1), 200.
2. Webster, F., Christian, J., Mansfield, E., Bhattacharyya, O., Hawker, G., Levinson, W., et al. (2015). Capturing the experiences of patients across multiple complex interventions: a meta-qualitative approach. *BMJ Open*, **5**:e007664.
3. Edwards, A., & Elwyn, G. (2009). *Shared Decision-Making in Health Care: Achieving Evidence-Based Patient Choice*. Oxford, Oxford University Press.
4. Elwyn, G., O'Connor, A., Stacey, D., Volk, R., Edwards, A., Coulter, A., et al. (2006). Developing a quality criteria framework for patient decision aids: online international Delphi consensus process. *BMJ*, **333**(7565), 417.
5. Elwyn, G., Scholl, I., Tietbohl, C., Mann, M., Edwards, A.G., Clay, C., et al. (2013). 'Many miles to go…': a systematic review of the implementation of patient decision support interventions into routine clinical practice. *BMC Medical Informatics and Decision Making*, **13**(2), 1.
6. Légaré, F., Ratté, S., Gravel, K., & Graham, I.D. (2008). Barriers and facilitators to implementing shared decision-making in clinical practice: update of a systematic review of health professionals' perceptions. *Patient Education and Counseling*, **73**(3), 526–535.
7. Durand, M.-A., Alam, S., Grande, S.W., & Elwyn, G. (2016). 'Much clearer with pictures': using community-based participatory research to design and test a Picture Option Grid for underserved patients with breast cancer. *BMJ Open*, **6**(2):e010008.
8. Hargraves, I., LeBlanc, A., Shah, N.D., & Montori, V.M. (2016). Shared decision making: the need for patient-clinician conversation, not just information. *Health Affairs*, **35**(4), 627–629.
9. Charon, R. (2001). Narrative medicine: a model for empathy, reflection, profession, and trust. *JAMA*, **286**(15), 1897–1902.
10. Ong, L.M., De Haes, J.C., Hoos, A.M., & Lammes, F.B. (1995). Doctor-patient communication: a review of the literature. *Social Science & Medicine*, **40**(7), 903–918.
11. Martin, D.J., Garske, J.P., & Davis, M.K. (2000). Relation of the therapeutic alliance with outcome and other variables: a meta-analytic review. *Journal of Consulting and Clinical Psychology*, **68**(3), 438.
12. Levenstein, J.H., McCracken, E.C., McWhinney, I.R., Stewart, M.A., & Brown, J.B. (1986). The patient-centred clinical method. 1. A model for the doctor-patient interaction in family medicine. *Family Practice*, **3**(1), 24–30.
13. Brown, J., Stewart, M., McCracken, E., McWhinney, I.R., & Levenstein, J. (1986). The patient-centred clinical method. 2. Definition and application. *Family Practice*, **3**(2), 75–79.
14. Liberati, E.G., Gorli, M., Moja, L., Galuppo, L., Ripamonti, S., & Scaratti, G. (2015). Exploring the practice of patient centered care: the role of ethnography and reflexivity. *Social Science & Medicine*, **133**, 45–52.
15. Miles, A., & Mezzich, J. (2011). The care of the patient and the soul of the clinic: person-centered medicine as an emergent model of modern clinical practice. *International Journal of Person Centered Medicine*, **1**(2), 207–222.

Chapter 7

16. Hamilton, D., Heaven, B., Thomson, R., Wilson, J., & Exley, C. (2016). Multidisciplinary team decision-making in cancer and the absent patient: a qualitative study. *BMJ Open*, 6(7):e012559

17. Elwyn, G., Wieringa, S., & Greenhalgh, T. (2016). Clinical encounters in the post-guidelines era. *BMJ*, **353**, i3200.

18. Taylor, S.J.C., Pinnock, H., Epiphaniou, E., Pearce, G., Parke, H.L., Schwappach, A., et al. (2014). A rapid synthesis of the evidence on interventions supporting self-management for people with long-term conditions: PRISMS – Practical systematic Review of Self-Management Support for long-term conditions. *Health Services and Delivery Research*, No. 2.53.

19. Greenhalgh, T. (2016). *Cultural Contexts of Health: The Use of Narrative Research in the Health Sector*. World Health Organization Health Evidence Network Series. Copenhangen, World Health Organization Regional Office for Europe.

20. Department of Health (2001). The Expert Patient: A New Approach to Chronic Disease Management for the 21st Century. Available from: http://webarchive.national archives.gov.uk/+/www.dh.gov.uk/en/Publicationsandstatistics/Publications/PublicationsPolicyandGuidance/DH_4006801 (last accessed 14 January 2017).

21. Lorig, K.R., & Holman, H.R. (2003). Self-management education: history, definition, outcomes, and mechanisms. *Annals of Behavioral Medicine*, **26**(1), 1–7.

22. Steinsbekk, A., Rygg, L., Lisulo, M., Rise, M.B., & Fretheim, A. (2012). Group based diabetes self-management education compared to routine treatment for people with type 2 diabetes mellitus. A systematic review with meta-analysis. *BMC Health Services Research*, **12**(1), 1.

23. Greenhalgh, T., Wherton, J., Sugarhood, P., Hinder, S., Procter, R., & Stones, R. (2013). What matters to older people with assisted living needs? A phenomenological analysis of the use and non-use of telehealth and telecare. *Social Science & Medicine (1982)*, **93**, 86–94.

24. Panagioti, M., Richardson, G., Murray, E., Rogers, A., Kennedy, A., Newman, S., et al. (2014). Reducing Care Utilisation through Self-Management Interventions (RECURSIVE): a systematic review and meta-analysis. *Health Services and Delivery Research*, No. 2.54.

25. Gately, C., Rogers, A., & Sanders, C. (2007). Re-thinking the relationship between long-term condition self-management education and the utilisation of health services. *Social Science & Medicine*, **65**(5), 934–945.

26. Caron-Flinterman, J.F., Broerse, J.E., & Bunders, J.F. (2005). The experiential knowledge of patients: a new resource for biomedical research? *Social Science & Medicine*, **60**(11), 2575–2584.

27. Snow, R., Humphrey, C., & Sandall, J. (2013). What happens when patients know more than their doctors? Experiences of health interactions after diabetes patient education: a qualitative patient-led study. *BMJ Open*, **3**(11):e003583.

28. May, C.R., Eton, D.T., Boehmer, K., Gallacher, K., Hunt, K., MacDonald, S., et al. (2014). Rethinking the patient: using Burden of Treatment Theory to understand the changing dynamics of illness. *BMC Health Services Research*, **14**(1), 1.

29. Vassilev, I., Rogers, A., Kennedy, A., & Koetsenruijter, J. (2014). The influence of social networks on self-management support: a metasynthesis. *BMC Public Health*, **14**(1), 1.

30. Health Foundation (2016). A Practical Guide to Self-Management Support. Available from: http://www.health.org.uk/publication/practical-guide-self-management-support (last accessed 14 January 2017).

31. Kendall, E., & Rogers, A. (2007). Extinguishing the social? State sponsored self-care policy and the Chronic Disease Self-Management Programme. *Disability & Society*, **22**(2), 129–143.

32. Hinder, S., & Greenhalgh, T. (2012). 'This does my head in'. Ethnographic study of self-management by people with diabetes. *BMC Health Services Research*, **12**(1), 83.

33. Shove, E., Pantzar, M., & Watson, M. (2012). *The Dynamics of Social Practice: Everyday Life and How it Changes*. London, Sage Publications.

34. Scott, I. (2009). What are the most effective strategies for improving quality and safety of health care? *Internal Medicine Journal*, **39**(6), 389–400.

35. Mockford, C., Staniszewska, S., Griffiths, F., & Herron-Marx, S. (2012). The impact of patient and public involvement on UK NHS health care: a systematic review. *International Journal for Quality in Health Care*, **24**(1), 28–38.

36. Greenhalgh, T., Humphrey, C., & Woodard, F. (2010). *User Involvement in Healthcare*. Oxford, John Wiley & Sons.

37. Litva, A., Canvin, K., Shepherd, M., Jacoby, A., & Gabbay, M. (2009). Lay perceptions of the desired role and type of user involvement in clinical governance. *Health Expectations*, **12**(1), 81–91.

38. Rise, M.B., Solbjør, M., Lara, M.C., Westerlund, H., Grimstad, H., & Steinsbekk, A. (2013). Same description, different values. How service users and providers define patient and public involvement in health care. *Health Expectations*, **16**(3), 266–276.

39. Nathan, S., Johnston, L., & Braithwaite, J. (2011). The role of community representatives on health service committees: staff expectations vs. reality. *Health Expectations*, **14**(3), 272–284.

40. Doherty, C., & Stavropoulou, C. (2012). Patients' willingness and ability to participate actively in the reduction of clinical errors: a systematic literature review. *Social Science & Medicine*, **75**(2), 257–263.

41. Bate, P., & Robert, G. (2007). *Bringing User Experience to Healthcare Improvement: The Concepts, Methods and Practices of Experience-Based Design*. Abingdon, Radcliffe Publishing.

Chapter 7

Chapter 8 **Technology**

8.1 The myth of technological determinism

By technology, I mean hardware and software (information and communication technologies or ICTs). In healthcare, such a definition would include a vast range of things, from smartphone apps and decision support systems through to electronic records, databases (big, small and in between) and the Internet. I want to narrow the scope of this chapter to examples of technologies that contain evidence or help us use evidence (as conventionally defined in the evidence-based healthcare (EBHC) literature). So what I am mainly talking about here is apps, decision support systems and other platforms that help either clinicians or patients access and/or apply research evidence. In Chapter 10, I will cover online peer support networks.

EBHC evolved in parallel with computer power in the 1990s and 2000s. The routine search for evidence to answer clinical questions became possible only because most research studies are electronically indexed on searchable databases accessible via the Internet. And most clinicians who are keen on EBHC are also what I would call technology savvy (some would say geeks). Partly for that reason, research into how to implement EBHC often involves someone developing and testing a technology.

In this section, I want to explode a myth: that the introduction of a technology can produce a particular outcome with any degree of predictability (an assumption known as *determinism*). If I prescribe a drug to a patient, I can predict with some confidence (e.g. using relative risk reduction or number needed to treat) whether and to what extent that drug will help them. If I offer them a technology (or provide a new technology to their clinician), the outcome cannot be predicted in the same way. This is an important principle that many academics and policymakers have yet to grasp.

Let me put my cards on the table: I think a lot of research done on technologies by EBHC geeks is very weak. Many such researchers are locked (naively and inappropriately) into the traditional hierarchy of evidence, so they consider the randomised controlled trial to be the pinnacle of high-quality evidence, just as it is when testing the efficacy of drugs. They thus design a technology-on versus technology-off trial – for example, of computer-based decision support versus paper-based guidelines. If they demonstrate a difference between the two arms of their trial, they claim that the technology 'works'. And if they do not demonstrate such a difference, they conclude it does not 'work'.

On one level, they would be correct, of course. But – as always with the implementation of software – the devil is in the sociotechnical detail [1]. What do I mean by sociotechnical? I mean that technologies have social meaning and are made to 'work' (if at all) through the wider network of people, other technologies, spaces and places that make up our lives. In other words, they are not plug and play.

A computerised decision support package, for example, will require the clinician to enter data into particular fields in a particular order (and, of course, the clinician must have access to a computer at the point of care). At a macro level, this package will require the organisation to have made a strategic decision to invest in a particular decision support package, install it on all of its computers and provide helpdesk and technical support for it. Built into the software will be numerous assumptions about the primary work tasks (who makes the clinical decision, when and with what information) and secondary work tasks (how the performance of the clinician will be assessed, how and by whom the work will be audited and billed and so on).

Anyone who has ever given their elderly relative a technology in the hope that it will make the relative's (and their own) life easier will know that technologies can generate problems as well as (or instead of) solving them. Technologies make cognitive and practical demands on us. They cost money. They need passwords. They take time to boot up. They freeze, crash and malfunction (in other words, the technology can become the patient). They may or may not be interoperable with other technologies on which a task depends. They lack flexibility (you can sit in the bath reading the paper version of the *Lancet* – but not the electronic version). And they have symbolic value – both positive (the smartphone symbolises connectedness, modernity, sophistication) and negative (a pendant alarm symbolises age, frailty, dependence).

Technologies can be socially and organisationally clunky. Any technology offered to patients (with a view to supporting self-management) or introduced into a healthcare organisation (with a view to changing how clinicians do their work) will require the intended user to make numerous changes – some subtle, some not so subtle – in the way they go about their everyday business. Furthermore, the introduction of a new technology will very often have unintended consequences for other people down the line (e.g. it might make work for the IT department).

Chapter 8

Don't get me wrong – I love technology. It has huge potential for getting evidence-based information to people who need it. But it is not the panacea people sometimes claim it is. It takes *work* and resources to implement a technology, to embed it into our lives and our workplaces and to deal with its unintended consequences. Too much research into the use of technologies to support evidence-based care has ignored the personal, social and organisational (not to mention the political and financial) dimensions, so I make no apology for giving these dimensions pride of place in this chapter.

The remainder of this chapter considers how we might explore the uptake and use (and the non-uptake and non-use) of technologies in the pursuit of evidence-based care. In Section 8.2, I look at apps, or what might be called 'lightweight' ICTs (easily downloaded, affordable, freestanding [2]) for both patients and clinicians. After that, I consider more 'heavyweight' technologies [2], such as Web-based portals and tools that are connected to a greater or lesser extent to other technologies and systems. In Sections 8.3 and 8.4, I cover the vexing question of why patients and clinicians, respectively, are so often reluctant to use the technologies we believe would support evidence-based management. In Section 8.5, I offer some tips for improving the uptake and use of technologies by both patients and clinicians.

8.2 Apps to support evidence-based (self-)management?

In this technological age, who has not downloaded an app with high hopes of making a mundane task quicker, more convenient or more fun? Quite a few people actually, so let us remember that those of us who do our shopping, banking, restaurant booking, international travel planning and evidence-based decision making with a few clicks on our smartphone are still in an elite minority. But before I consider people who cannot or will not use apps (the 'digitally excluded'), let me share a few examples of what is currently available to those who do.

To find an example to work through, I went on to one of several websites offering reviews of medical apps (www.imedicalapps.com) and downloaded its 'Medical App of the Month', which happened to be a statin intolerance tool from the American College of Cardiologists. It was free, based on the kind of evidence that makes it into Cochrane reviews and relevant to me as I had a relative who was wondering if his muscle pains and general tiredness were due to his statin tablets. The app was easy to use, and whilst the algorithm took me down one or two cul-de-sacs of the screamingly obvious ('determine if patient has done anything [to cause muscle pain] such as moving furniture'), it did remind me of some questions to ask him, listed potentially interacting medications and reminded me of some comorbidities that could increase the likelihood of intolerance.

Entering some individual data on to the app did not tell me whether my relative's muscle pains were due to the statin, or indeed whether this drug should be discontinued, but it did alert me quickly and painlessly to some evidence-based actions that could be taken to progress this case (adjusting other medication, treating comorbidities, an additional blood test) – all within a few seconds of first opening the app. It also taught me a lot in the process of using it. My relative took some of the information (copied on to a bit of paper) to start a conversation with his doctor.

The statin intolerance app 'worked' for five reasons. First, I am already a user of medical apps. Downloading them and fiddling with them is something I am trained to do and fits seamlessly into my life and work. Second, I already own the technology needed to host the app (a smartphone), and nothing was preventing me from downloading it (this is not always true when trying to download software on to what is technically termed the 'locked-down environment' of an organisational computer network). Third, I consider the app to be evidence-based (because I know and trust the professional organisation that produced it). Fourth, my relative (who is not tech-savvy) did not need to do anything with the technology because I was helping him. Fifth, I did not need to breach confidentiality, since the app did not ask me for the person's name, date of birth or any other identifying information. In short, this was a good example of how carefully selected medical apps can work well in clinical care.

Another area where medical apps appear to work well is in clinical education. My son, currently a final-year medical student (and, of course, a tech-savvy smartphone user), uses dozens of apps to learn everything from human anatomy to the assessment of chest pain. He also has apps for helping make diagnoses, revising and practising for exams, and pretending to be the patient so he can (virtually) 'examine' them.

Once you have been on a course in basic programming, apps are not hard to build. Small wonder that there are now well over 100 000 medical and health apps on the market [3]. Whilst my son and other students and junior doctors like him are convinced that the apps on their smartphones save them time and improve their practice, there is remarkably little hard evidence on who uses medical apps, for what, to what benefit and at what risk [3,4]. Indeed, the field is so fast-moving that any survey of such questions would be out of date before it was published. One interesting recent study found that the vast majority of mobile app use by junior doctors happened when they were not on duty, suggesting that there is more to be done to integrate such apps with point-of-care decision-making in practice [5].

The main problem with medical apps is quality control. Just because an app claims to be evidence-based does not mean it is [6]. Worryingly, a recent review of insulin dosing apps intended for use by patients with diabetes concluded that most of them 'provide no protection against, and may actively contribute to, incorrect or inappropriate dose recommendations that put current users at risk of both catastrophic overdose and more subtle harms resulting from suboptimal glucose control' [7]. Whatever you have heard, there is no app-driven technological revolution happening in diabetes management.

Most medical apps do *not* hold the kitemark of a pukka professional body, and many if not most are marketed (or given away) by someone with a conflict of interest. Would you use a statin intolerance app that was made by the manufacturer of a statin, for example? There has been much talk of whether medical apps should be formally appraised, approved and regulated [8]. The US Food and Drug Administration (FDA) [9], European Commission [10] and UK Medicines and Healthcare Devices Regulatory Agency [11] have tried (with partial success). But (to borrow a title from an editorial Tony Delamothe once wrote for the *British Medical Journal* on regulating the content of websites) such a task has been likened to an attempt to kitemark the west wind – that is, it is likely to prove practically, techologically and legally impossible.

One of the fastest-growing areas of e-health research is in apps designed to support self-management of chronic disease by patients. The range of such apps is already vast, and randomised trials of their effectiveness in improving disease outcomes are becoming common. The most widely researched conditions in this genre are diabetes (in which improvements have been shown in blood glucose control but not in weight loss, mood, emotional well-being or quality of life with the use of self-management apps) [12] and asthma (in which self-management tasks, medication use and quality of life seemed to improve with the use of an app, but there was no consistent benefit on symptom control or markers of disease severity) [13].

A more recent review broadly confirmed these findings for diabetes and asthma, and also found limited evidence of benefit from patient self-management apps in cardiovascular disease [14]. Again, this is a fast-moving field, and I have no doubt that in future editions of this book, this paragraph will require extensive updating.

But before we get carried away doing more trials to determine the influence of 'app' versus 'no app' in primary outcome A and secondary outcomes B, C and D in disease X, I want to question the fundamental basis of such research. I share the concern of medical sociologist Deborah Lupton, who considers health and medical apps not merely as containers of evidence (or not), but also as *cultural artefacts* – that is, 'digital objects that are the products of human decision-making, underpinned by tacit assumptions, norms and discourses already circulating in the social and cultural contexts in which they are generated, marketed and used' [3].

In other words, apps contain inbuilt assumptions about what matters to us, what choices we might wish to make, what skills and knowledge we have (or lack) and how we will act. In Section 7.3, I described self-management as a social practice (i.e. a whole way of life, not merely a set of technical tasks such as measuring one's blood glucose and administering medication). Nowhere is that more true than in our dietary choices – and therein lies a tale.

I once agreed (against my better judgement) to join a group of enthusiastic young doctors who were applying for funding to test the impact of an app on the progression of non-alcoholic fatty liver disease (NAFLD) in Bangladeshis. Thankfully, we did not get the money, but the flawed line of reasoning to which I once added my name is a good illustration of what is wrong with the fashion of developing apps intended to change patient behaviour.

I am no expert on NAFLD (although my co-applicants were). As I understand it, the condition is caused by a build-up of fat in the liver in people who are overweight and continue to consume more energy than they are expending. It is associated with high cholesterol levels and it predisposes to diabetes and heart attack. In a sense, a diagnosis of NAFLD (made by a blood test and liver scan) is a marker for a lifestyle that is getting dangerously close to doing permanent damage. And it is common in people of Bangladeshi origin who live in the United Kingdom.

The research evidence on how to treat NAFLD appears to be strong [15]. The cornerstone is modification of lifestyle – most especially dietary intake. Specifically, someone with NAFLD needs to eat smaller portions of almost everything and ensure that their diet is high in fruits, vegetables and protein but low in fat, sugar and salt.

An app to convey this evidence to patients was the brainchild of a bright young doctor working in a liver unit whose outpatient clinics were increasingly booked up by Bangladeshi patients with NAFLD. The idea was that when a patient was contemplating a meal, they could enter data into the app and receive a score for how well it aligned with evidence-based dietary recommendations. The information in the app could be translated into the relevant ethnic languages.

The idea was rightly bounced by the grant committee. Even though we had offered to seek patient input into the design of the app, there was no getting round the fact that the whole idea was predicated on the assumptions that (i) people make their dietary choices in a rational way (they don't – eating is a social practice that is strongly influenced by cultural tastes and expectations [16]); (ii) giving people an app would mean that they would use it (not true – you can lead a horse to water but you can't necessarily make them drink); and (iii) the main issue the patients needed help with was the technical task of assessing the nutritional value of food rather than the socioemotional one of navigating the food-based practices and hospitality rituals in South Asian culture (again, not true – as Bente Halkier found in her study of Pakistani families in Denmark [17] and Sue Hinder and myself found in our UK study of living with diabetes [18]).

In sum, apps to support evidence-based decision-making by clinicians and evidence-based self-management by patients hold much promise – but they also bring risks and challenges. My advice is summarised in the ten questions in Box 8.1.

Box 8.1 Ten questions to ask of a medical or health app

These questions are designed to be used to assess apps aimed at clinicians, patients or the lay public. They are not a definitive or universal list and may need to be adapted to suit different purposes.

1 On what evidence is it based – and is this evidence (i) relevant, (ii) complete and up to date and (iii) robust?

2 Who is selling it? What are their values and conflicts of interest? If they are giving it away, why?

3 How easy is it to use? Is there a helpdesk facility or other troubleshooting options?

4 Who developed/designed it, and for what purpose? What assumptions did they make about patient and/or clinician behaviour and are these justified? Were intended users of the app involved in its design?

5 What other technologies (e.g. smartphone) are needed to make the app work? Does it work on all possible platforms? Does it need to interface with other software, and if so, which? Is it accessible when you need it (e.g. does it need a good wifi signal)?

6 What people (e.g. nurse, carer) are needed to use the app, and what training/ skills do they need? Is the use of this app going to alter current practices and/or generate work for someone?

7 What are the risks or unintended consequences of using the app?

8 What data does the app ask for? What happens to data entered onto it? Does this meet relevant security/privacy standards?

9 What country or setting was the app designed for, and to what extent do the assumptions on which is it based transfer to your country/ setting?

10 How much does the app cost to (i) buy and (ii) implement (and is it worth it)? Is it freestanding or linked to the purchase of other products or services? How do alternatives (technological and non-technological) compare?

8.3 Why do patients resist technologies?

As I observed in Section 8.1, EBHC enthusiasts are often at the geeky end of the spectrum. They design technologies to help implement evidence, then cannot understand why other people (patients, fellow clinicians) do not share their enthusiasm. In this section, I will consider the patient perspective.

In a paper bravely entitled, 'Why Didn't It Work?', Annie Lau and colleagues described their experiences with Healthy.me, which is what they call a 'personally controlled health management system' for asthma, consisting of a personal health record (not linked to their clinician's record) [19]. The various elements of the package – including a personal asthma management plan, a forum for online peer support, online well-being support programmes and an internal email system for access to clinicians by the self-managing patient – had been shown in randomised trials to improve outcomes for asthma.

On the face of it, the Healthy.me technology cleverly bundled much of what works in asthma care into a single, well-designed website that was free at the point of use. The authors constructed their hypothesis as follows: compared to those offered usual care, people randomised to the web-based personally controlled health-management system would be:

- more likely to obtain or update a written asthma action plan;
- more likely to make planned visits to a healthcare professional for asthma;
- less likely to make unplanned visits to a healthcare professional for asthma;
- less likely to experience deterioration in their asthma (as measured by acute exacerbations, ongoing poor control, need for up-titration of medication or loss of work/school days).

What could possibly go wrong? Answer: almost nobody used the web portal. More than 80% of the 154 patients assigned to the intervention arm of the trial either did not access the website at all or did so only once. Whilst the authors faithfully applied their predefined statistical tests to compare the participants in the technology-on arm of the study with those in the technology-off arm (on an intention-to-treat basis), the findings meant little compared to the colossal non-adoption rate, and differences between the two arms of the trial were not statistically significant.

To their credit, the authors assessed users' perceptions of the technology using the validated Technology Acceptance Model (whose main dimensions are usefulness and ease of use [20]) and sought reasons from those who did not use it. People who used the technology found it moderately easy to use and moderately useful in managing their asthma. But the qualitative (free-text) data reported in the paper suggest that non-users (the overwhelming majority) saw little advantage in the web-based system and did not feel that the effort required was worth it, especially given the many competing demands on their time. The authors concluded:

> Consumers must perceive the need for assistance with a task and assign priority to the task supported by the eHealth intervention. Additionally, the cost of adopting the intervention (e.g. additional effort, time spent learning the new system) must be lower than the benefit. [19]

In Section 2.4, I summarised research by Everett Rogers and colleagues on the attributes of innovations, and pointed out that the single most important attribute is relative advantage. As the study of Healthy.me illustrates, relative advantage is not an intrinsic property of the innovation but in the eye of the potential adopter. If he or she cannot see the benefit of using it, he or she will be very unlikely to even try.

As I emphasised in Section 7.3, living with chronic illness involves far more than completion of a set of biomedical tasks. Self-management technologies tend to be designed around a typical, idealised (and somewhat stereotypical) patient and are oriented to supporting and monitoring the more biomedical aspects of management (in the previous example, getting a written asthma management plan, visiting the doctor or nurse and appearing – or not – in the emergency department). The free-text comments by participants in the Healthy.me trial describe a much wider range of issues and activities impacting on their asthma (e.g. the competing priority of looking after other sick family members). Not only did the technology not help them with these issues, it sometimes interfered with them, because it took significant time and effort.

Note that in most trials, only people prepared to use a technology will get as far as being randomised, which explains why there are dozens of examples of technologies that were shown to 'work' in randomised trials but flopped when rolled out in the real world.

In sum, patients have their reasons – often good ones – for not using the technologies we have carefully built to make their care more evidence-based. If this is the end result of your efforts, try not to blame the patient. Go back to the drawing board – but first, find yourself a diverse group of patients and invite them to be partners in the design process (see Section 6.4 for a general overview of co-designing research *with* patients as opposed to doing research *on* patients).

I have been involved in a number of technology co-design projects myself, most recently one led by my senior research fellow Joe Wherton. The first step of such a process is to undertake detailed ethnographic studies 'in the wild' – in other words, in people's homes (and shopping centres, workplaces, pubs, betting shops and anywhere else they are prepared to allow you to research their lives) [21]. Only when you have done enough qualitative research to understand what really matters to people and how their illness plays out in the context of family, neighbourhood, community and so on will you begin to be able to design a 'patient-centred' technology.

The second phase of technology co-design involves bringing patients, carers, clinicians and technology designers together to discuss key scenarios (derived from your qualitative work) and consider how the technology might be designed or redesigned to deal with those scenarios [22]. Expect to see mismatches of perspective between these different groups, and be prepared to facilitate lively discussion.

The final phase is development and piloting of the technology in real-world settings.

'Where is the randomised trial in this sequence?', you may ask. The answer is, I am not sure it is needed. Before you attack me for promoting methods that are too far down the hierarchy of evidence for your standards, let me direct you to a blog by Enrico Coiera, one of the world's leading professors of health informatics (and the author of one of the best books on that subject [23]). In his blog, Enrico analyses the success of the Pokémon Go game, which rapidly attracted millions of users and succeeded (where public health programmes had so often failed) in getting the 'sofa generation' out on to the streets, taking exercise. He comments:

> While healthcare researchers are slowly coming to grips with 'new' ideas like gamification and social media to defeat obesity, the game industry has jumped the queue and may have already done it. Silicon valley has drawn down on its deep well of expertise in building large and complex software systems, and in embedding such systems into the real world. They have drawn on their deep experience with and understanding of the psychology of online social media, of what makes games 'fun', and what makes them 'sticky'.
>
> I doubt if Niantic, the Pokemon company, looked to randomized clinical trials to design and implement their system. The world of software moves too fast for that. It has an engineering culture of fail early, fail often. And because of that, it has as much right as scientists to claim that it is driven by experimentation and data, or as the philosopher Karl Popper would have said, conjecture and refutation.

In short, when producing technologies that are usable and which motivate people to use them, the software industry knows a thing or two. Design links to both a science (engineering) and the arts (creativity, aesthetics), but is more than a simple intersection between the two. It sits on a very different shelf in the academic library from the randomised trials beloved by epidemiologists and clinicians [24]. I am not claiming that we should abandon trials of technologies in patient self-management and related activities altogether, but I am saying that the EBHC community has much to learn from methodologies employed by other academic disciplines and by the commercial sector. Given the continuing enthusiasm of research funders for randomised trial designs of technologies, I think it is time to ask whether EBHC's beloved hierarchy of evidence is holding back progress in this particular field.

8.4 Why do clinicians resist technologies?

This section is based loosely on a report my team produced for the UK National Institute for Health Research (NIHR) on why non-adoption and abandonment by clinicians seems to stymie the introduction of so many new technologies in healthcare [25]. In that report, we cited claims by others that 50–80% of new ICT systems in healthcare fail. I never tracked down the original data on which that claim was based, and I suspect it is apocryphal. Nevertheless, I also suspect that the estimate is not wildly out. As Rodriguez and Pozzebon said a few years ago:

> Most [healthcare ICT] implementations fail because, despite high investments in terms of both time and financial resources, physicians simply do not use them. [26]

In Section 7.2, I addressed the topic of implementing evidence with patients in the clinical encounter. Much of that section was about the computer-based tools being developed for shared decision-making with patients. Indeed, I wondered whether to put it under Chapter 7 (Patients) or this chapter (Technologies). In the end, I decided to discuss the *potential* for such tools in the chapter on patients and to consider here an equally important issue: the fact that such tools are rarely *actually* used in the clinical encounter.

In 2013, Glyn Elwyn and colleagues published a systematic review of clinicians' use of tools to involve patients in clinical decisions [27]. They found many evidence-based tools (some of which are described in Section 7.2) but very limited uptake by frontline clinicians. They describe this lack of uptake as due to 'clinical inertia', which they attribute in turn to a 'lack of confidence in the content of decision support interventions and concern about disruption to established workflows, ultimately contributing to organizational inertia regarding their adoption' (p. 14).

The expression 'clinical inertia' aligns broadly with the widely used terms 'lack of clinical engagement' and 'clinician resistance' – and implies on the surface that the fault lies with the (Luddite, obtuse, incurious) personality of the clinician. But as Elwyn et al. go on to say, the clinicians' resistance has two upstream causes: *concerns about the quality of the evidence* (and the recommendations derived from them) and *inability to integrate the use of the tool with existing work practices.* Their conclusion, although expressed in somewhat vague terms, resonates with a wider body of literature on the introduction of ICTs in organisations.

The discovery over 50 years ago that technologies, whilst creating opportunities, often require us to change our work practices was the basis of an important (but, sadly, often overlooked) set of 'principles for sociotechnical design' summarised by Albert Cherns in the 1970s and updated in the 1980s [28,29]. Chris Clegg extended and improved on these principles in 2000, increasing the number from 10 to 19 [30]. In Box 8.2, I offer a revised set of principles, based on the work of all these authors, but omitting much of Clegg's added detail for simplicity.

Perhaps the most important principle of sociotechnical design is the first one given in Box 8.2 – that introducing technologies in an organisation is a *social* process that depends on values, mindsets and engagement. It is, furthermore, an evolutionary process (sociotechnical systems are *grown*, not *built*, and the metaphor of an ecosystem is a useful one). What this means is that if you seek to introduce a new technology into your organisation or department, the 'soft' elements of organisational change (opening up a space for dialogue, listening to concerns, allowing people time to argue out the challenges – see Section 5.5) are central, not marginal, to the project's success. The best people to design the new activities and workflows are the people who live and breathe the existing ones. And so on.

The tenth principle in Box 8.2 reminds us that introducing new technology is a *political* process (political with a small 'p', meaning 'to do with power'). In 1983, Lynne Markus published a paper on workplace resistance to new IT systems that has since become a classic, entitled 'Power, Politics and Information Systems' [31]. She divided resistance into three types of factor:

1. **People-determined:** Personalities, goals, capabilities and so on.
2. **System-determined:** Features of the technology and how it is implemented.
3. **Interactional or 'sociotechnical':** To do with the interactions between people and technologies.

One of the points made by Markus is that introducing a technology inevitably changes who holds the power. For example, when medical records were paper-based, few people ever looked at them except clinicians and the occasional auditor. Now that many medical records are electronic, and based

---

Box 8.2 Principles of sociotechnical design

Sociotechnical design is the development and adaptation of work processes alongside the development, introduction and customisation of technology.

Meta-principles

1 Sociotechnical design is a social process in which values, mindsets and engagement are critical.

2 Design should reflect the needs of patients, staff and the service as a whole.

Content principles

3 Design entails multiple task allocations between and amongst humans and technologies.

4 No more should be specified than is absolutely essential, and what is essential should be made explicit.

5 Core processes should be integrated.

6 As far as possible, problems should be dealt with at source (e.g. feed local data back to local teams in a timely way).

Process principles

7 People should be involved in designing the jobs they are to perform.

8 Resources and support are required for design.

9 Evaluation and group learning are integral to the design process.

10 System design involves political processes; attention needs to be paid to power dynamics.

Source: Adapted from Cherns [28,29] and Clegg [30].

---

increasingly on coded data, it is much easier for managers to study the work of clinicians by converting the clinical and administrative codes into metrics of activity. If you are a clinician who does not want managers breathing down your neck, you might resist the introduction of electronic records. The managers are also playing a political hand (if they get the data on doctors' work activity they might be able to performance-manage them in particular directions), with good reason to push for greater digitisation of records.

In such situations, subtle power games will be played, and the different players are unlikely to make their real motives explicit [32]. Doctors will talk in terms of 'protecting patient confidentiality' and managers in terms of 'modernisation'. Because of the political undercurrents, approaches to overcoming resistance need to be directed at their underlying causes, not at the excuses people give when asked. For example, if resistance is 'people-determined', solutions will take the form of education, incentives and hands-on participation sessions; if 'system-determined', solutions lie in better technical design (including human factors research – see Pascale Carayon's work on how to do this in healthcare [33,34]). But if, as is usually the case, the roots of resistance are at the more political end of the sociotechnical spectrum, solutions will be more complex and lie in improving organisational work-flows, redressing power dynamics and the like.

A classic case study of sociotechnical problems in a hospital was described by Symon and colleagues in 1996 [35]. A new electronic record system was so unpopular that work almost ground to a halt. Qualitative research surfaced the underlying problem: inscribed into the software was a host of (incorrect) assumptions about how work happened – and if the electronic system was used, people simply could not keep the show on the road. The authors commented:

> Work processes can be described in two ways: the way things are **supposed to work** and the way they **do work**. Software that is designed to support standard procedures can be too brittle. [35]

The interdisciplinary academic field of computer-supported cooperative work (CSCW) studies how groups of people use ICTs to collaborate on work projects. A central focus of this research is the gap between how things are supposed to work and how they actually do work. CSCW researchers talk about *articulation work* (sometimes colloquially known as 'workarounds'), which they define as:

> carrying through a course of action despite local contingencies, unantici-pated glitches, incommensurable opinions and beliefs or inadequate knowledge of local circumstances. [36]

If we are to improve the dismal success rate of ICTs in healthcare, we need to find better ways of studying the process of articulation and exploring how the principles of sociotechnical design (Box 8.2) are applied in practice. As Wanda Pratt and her colleagues emphasise in a paper entitled 'Incorporating Ideas from Computer-Supported Cooperative Work' [37], this will usually comprise a parallel process of supporting staff and patients to (re)design care processes and at the same time refining and customising the technologies that support those processes to make them less 'clunky' in practice. Note that sociotechnical design is not a technical and rational process that you can drive using a checklist but a *social and creative* process in which people listen to each other, work together, try things out and collectively muddle through.

I have argued elsewhere for the greater use of ethnography to illuminate the sociotechnical work of implementing ICTs in organisations [38]. In that paper, I describe a study by Yong Han and colleagues, published in the *Journal of the American medical Association* [39]. These authors set out to demonstrate in a large, quasi-experimental before-and-after study that mortality in a paediatric tertiary care centre (dealing with very sick children, often transferred as emergencies from other centres) would be reduced by the introduction of a computerised physician order entry (CPOE) system to support safer prescribing and dispensing of medication.

To the authors' surprise (since the CPOE system was 'evidence-based' – that is, built around what was known to make prescribing safer), mortality increased significantly (from 2.80 to 6.57%) after the system was introduced. The authors, whose paper otherwise follows the experimental and quantitative style typical of biomedical papers, explain these unexpected findings thus [39]:

> *The usual chain of events that occurred when a patient was admitted through our transport system was altered after CPOE implementation. Before implementation of CPOE, after radio contact with the transport team, the ICU [intensive care unit] fellow was allowed to order critical medications/drips, which then were prepared by the bedside ICU nurse in anticipation of patient arrival. When needed, the ICU fellow could also make arrangements for the patient to receive an emergent diagnostic imaging study before coming into the ICU. A full set of admission orders could be written and ready before patient arrival. After CPOE implementation, order entry was not allowed until after the patient had physically arrived to the hospital and been fully registered into the system, leading to potential delays in new therapies and diagnostic testing (this policy later was rectified). The physical process of entering stabilization orders often required an average of ten clicks on the computer mouse per order, which translated to 1 to 2 minutes per single order as compared with a few seconds previously needed to place the same order by written form. Because the vast majority of computer terminals were linked to the hospital computer system via wireless signal, communication bandwidth was often exceeded during peak operational periods, which created additional delays between each click on the computer mouse. Sometimes the computer screen seemed frozen. (pp. 1508–1509)*

This honest account offers some important empirical and methodological lessons. Empirically, the commercial CPOE system (which had been extensively tested before release) did not perform as anticipated in real-world situations for three reasons. First, assumptions, constraints and access privileges which had been built into (or, to use the term preferred by sociologists, 'inscribed in') the technology as well-intentioned safety features could not be over-ridden to meet local contingencies, even when a child's life was at stake. Second, system designers missed critical elements of the collaborative work routine (input of key staff in a particular, time-dependent sequence) for emergency admission. Third, electronic processes ran an order of magnitude more slowly than their written or spoken equivalent.

Methodologically, this CPOE example shows that even relatively crude real-life observations presented in narrative form can convey much about the interaction between the material properties of technologies, time, place, space and human action and interaction in the complex and fast-paced world of emergency healthcare. It suggests that even richer insights could be generated by applying more sophisticated techniques of qualitative observation: for example, if detailed ethnographic field notes (what anthropologists call 'thick description') were made; if these observational field notes were supplemented with video or screen-capture technologies; or if talk were recorded, transcribed and analysed to facilitate study of the subtle complexities of interaction between humans and technologies. In other words, we could learn a lot from ethnography.

In my view, if we are to illuminate why such a high proportion of technology projects fail in healthcare (and reduce that proportion), we need fewer randomised trials of technologies and more in-depth qualitative research in the real world. My colleague and co-author Dr Deborah Swinglehurst has led some excellent ethnographic research studies on the complex sociotechnical interactions that both explain successes and account for failures when healthcare teams seek to use technologies to support evidence-based care in chronic disease management [40] and repeat prescribing [41].

The examples I have given so far in this section relate to medium-scale technologies introduced into a single organisation. I have spent a significant proportion of my research career studying attempts to introduce large-scale technological innovation at a regional or national level [1,42,43]. To avoid making this section unmanageably long, I will not describe that work in detail here – but I will say that whatever problems happen at the meso (organisational) level seem to be even more likely to happen if the project is expanded beyond a single organisation. Box 8.3 shows a summary of the lessons I learnt from evaluating England's National Programme for IT, which I produced for Bob Wachter when he was leading a review of healthcare IT for the Department of Health in 2016.

I discuss the sociotechnical perspective further in Section 11.3 when I talk about actor-networks.

8.5 Ten tips for using technologies to support EBHC

1. Get real about where you lie on the geek spectrum

If there is a recurring tip through this book, it is that EBHC keenies should get out more. In Section 8.1 I gently suggested that people who are keen on EBHC are significantly geekier than the rest of the universe. (I can say that because I am pretty geeky myself). Remember that, statistically speaking, most of the people whose lives you want to improve with your evidence-based gadget are less enthused by technology than you are.

> **Box 8.3 Ten things I learnt about 'heavy' ICT from evaluating England's National Programme for IT**
>
> 1 The bigger it is, the harder it gets.
> 2 Different stakeholders see things differently. There are six 'worlds':
>   a **Political:** The technology is a vehicle for delivering policy.
>   b **Clinical:** The technology is a tool to support professional practice.
>   c **Personal (patient/carer):** My data, my record.
>   d **Technical:** The technology is an elegant and useful design.
>   e **Commercial:** The technology is a means for delivering return on investment.
>   f **Legal/regulatory:** The technology is a potential can of information governance worms.
> 3 IT systems must be grown, not built (→ sociotechnical systems theory).
> 4 Tensions and paradoxes are inherent: they can be managed, but not resolved.
> 5 Knowledge is more than what gets passed up the line.
> 6 'Hard' approaches (goals/metrics/project management) must be balanced with 'soft' ones (debate/dialogue/collective sense-making).
> 7 Technical developers should be alert to the subtleties of clinical work and the realities of the NHS.
> 8 'Clinical engagement' is more about being listened to than being written to.
> 9 Much depends on frontline staff, who usually want to do a good job.
> 10 Government is respectfully reminded that:
>   a You can't contract for creativity.
>   b Civil servants don't have to drive the boat.
>   c Privacy is not a footnote.
>
> *Source: Summarised for policymakers from academic publications* [1,42,46].

2. Move beyond technological determinism

If you think that introducing a technology will 'cause' people to behave in a particular way, you are a naive technological determinist – and, as such, you are a danger to any sensible change effort. Read Section 8.1 and try to understand why technologies should be thought of as tools for supporting change but *not* as drivers of change.

3. Stop and think before designing an app

Every young clinician these days wants to have a line on their CV that they designed an app to educate their colleagues, empower their patients or disseminate the findings of a research study. But before you add your contribution to the haystack of 'lightweight ICTs' from which the rest of us will need to extract the needles of useful technologies, read Section 8.2 and study

Box 8.1. Your app does not merely need to encode some evidence-based information. It also needs to add value to what is already available and fit seamlessly into people's lives, lifestyles and work practices. Stop thinking about your app for a moment; start thinking about the people who might use it, the context in which they might use it and the (intended and unintended) consequences of their using it.

4. Learn more about how patients live with illness

If you want to develop technological solutions for patients, first get your head round the problem you are setting out to solve. In Section 7.5, I suggested you learn what illness means to patients. This tip is in the same vein. If you are living with illness yourself (or have a close relative with one), you will know that your (their) day-to-day activities and priorities do not map to the imagined life of the 'textbook patient'. The person who is ill will use technologies – but probably not the ones their doctor or nurse thinks they use, or in the way they imagine the technology *should* be used. Start with the real world; build on that.

5. Take randomised trials of technology-on versus technology-off with a pinch of salt

It is still very fashionable in healthcare research (and in some – although, mercifully, not all – research funding panels) to view the randomised trial as the methodological gold standard whatever the research question and however important it is to capture the influence of context. If you have read and understood the work of the founding fathers (*sic*) of evidence-based medicine, this is not what Dave Sackett and his colleagues meant when they encouraged the use of randomised trials [44]. A randomised trial will tell you if technology A (version x.x used when the trial began n years ago) compared with technology B or no technology influenced outcome C in setting D at time T1–T2. Whether the trial shows a positive impact or not on its primary outcome, the result won't tell you whether the current version (y.y) of technology A is going to have a significant influence on outcome P in setting Q at time T3–T4 (apologies for the geek-speak).

6. Read more about design

In this chapter, I have only been able to skim the surface of the principles of design. In Section 8.3, I offered some references on technology co-design with patients. I also referred in passing to a great book by Nigel Cross called Designerly Ways of Knowing [24]. I strongly recommend you get hold of it and take the first steps on a journey into this fascinating discipline.

7. Study tasks and processes in organisations

Appendix A lists some approaches to process mapping – that is, unpacking the complex activities and interactions that make up clinical and administrative work in healthcare organisations. Once you start observing, in intimate detail, what people do, how they communicate and collaborate, and what role technologies play in this process, you will approach the introduction of technology with far greater wisdom.

A particularly useful aspect of studying tasks and processes is learning from workarounds. We need to shift from a view that in an ideal world technology works perfectly all the time to a view that acknowledges the messiness of the real world and the inevitable gap between any model of reality and reality itself (Paul Dourish and Genevieve Bell have written a wonderful book about this topic [45]). Workarounds may, by definition, be unofficial, but they are a feature of every sociotechnical system. They are what keeps the show on the road – and also a great source of learning about how to improve technologies and how we use them.

8. Take a course in ethnography

Ethnography was once the province of anthropologists, who travelled to far-off islands and donned a pith helmet to study the natives. These days, anthropologists are more likely to be found on hospital wards, in operating theatres or in the waiting rooms of GP surgeries, studying clinicians and patients in their natural habitats. Ethnography is not just a fancy name for standing around watching the world go by. It is a legitimate social science methodology that can be done well or badly. If you want to do the kind of research that involves studying technologies in organisations, a short course in ethnography would be a very good foundation.

9. Learn, and apply, the principles of sociotechnical design in organisations

Study the principles in Box 8.2. In their original (longer) form, these principles have stood the test of time. Designing and redesigning the microsystems for using technology in organisations is a social process, so make sure you involve people in it. Don't overspecify what needs to be done, either by the technology or by the people you think are going to use it. Let people on the front line work creatively to adapt processes and introduce technologies *their* way. Anticipate power struggles – and facilitate individuals and groups to work through them.

10. If you want technology-supported change, resource it

The introduction of a technology costs money. Not only do people need to be trained to use it, they need time out to argue about *whether* they need to use it, negotiate *how* they're going to use it and develop *workarounds* for keeping the show on the road despite it. The technology may save work for one group of people but it can still make work for another. A 'heavyweight' technology will have knock-ons for the wider IT system in the organisation – and hence for helpdesk support. Upgrades are rarely free. In short, you will need a budget to buy the technology, a budget to support its introduction and adoption, and a recurrent budget to support its continuing use.

References

1. Greenhalgh, T., Stramer, K., Bratan, T., Byrne, E., Russell, J., Hinder, S., & Potts, H. (2010). The devil's in the detail: final report of the independent evaluation of the Summary Care Record and HealthSpace programmes. London, University College London.
2. Bygstad, B. (2016). Generative innovation: a comparison of lightweight and heavyweight IT. *Journal of Information Technology*, doi:10.1057/jit.2016.15.
3. Lupton, D. (2014). Apps as artefacts: towards a critical perspective on mobile health and medical apps. *Societies*, 4(4), 606–622.
4. Ozdalga, E., Ozdalga, A., & Ahuja, N. (2012). The smartphone in medicine: a review of current and potential use among physicians and students. *Journal of Medical Internet Research*, **14**(5), e128.
5. Patel, R., Green, W., Shahzad, M.W., & Larkin, C. (2015). Use of mobile clinical decision support software by junior doctors at a UK teaching hospital: identification and evaluation of barriers to engagement. *JMIR mHealth and uHealth*, 3(3), e80.
6. Buijink, A., Visser, B.J., & Marshall, L. (2013). Medical apps for smartphones: lack of evidence undermines quality and safety. *Evidence Based Medicine*, **18**(3), 90–92.
7. Huckvale, K., Adomaviciute, S., Prieto, J.T., Leow, M.K.-S., & Car, J. (2015). Smartphone apps for calculating insulin dose: a systematic assessment. *BMC Medicine*, **13**(1), 1.
8. Kamerow, D. (2013). Regulating medical apps: which ones and how much? *BMJ*, **347**, f6009.
9. Yetisen, A.K., Martinez-Hurtado, J., da Cruz Vasconcellos, F., Simsekler, M.E., Akram, M.S., & Lowe, C.R. (2014). The regulation of mobile medical applications. *Lab on a Chip*, **14**(5), 833–840.
10. European Commission (2016). Guidelines on the Qualification and Classification of Stand Alone Software Used in Healthcare within the Regulatory Framework of Medical Devices. MEDDEV 2.1/6. Brussels, European Commission (DG Internal Market, Industry, Entrepreneurship and SMEs Directorate Consumer, Environmental and Health Technologies Unit Health Technology and Cosmetics).
11. Medicines and Healthcare Devices Regulatory Agency (2016). Guidance: Medical Device Stand-alone Software Including Apps (Including IVDMDs). Available from: https://www.gov.uk/government/uploads/system/uploads/attachment_data/file/549127/Software_flow_chart_Ed_1-01.pdf (last accessed 14 January 2017).
12. Pal, K., Eastwood, S.V., Michie, S., Farmer, A., Barnard, M.L., Peacock, R., et al. (2014). Computer-based interventions to improve self-management in adults

Chapter 8

with type 2 diabetes: a systematic review and meta-analysis. *Diabetes Care*, **37**(6), 1759–1766.

13. Morrison, D., Wyke, S., Agur, K., Cameron, E.J., Docking, R.I., MacKenzie, A.M., et al. (2014). Digital asthma self-management interventions: a systematic review. *Journal of Medical Internet Research*, **16**(2), e51.

14. Whitehead, L., & Seaton, P. (2016). The effectiveness of self-management mobile phone and tablet apps in long-term condition management: a systematic review. *Journal of Medical Internet Research*, **18**(5), e97.

15. Vernon, G., Baranova, A., & Younossi, Z. (2011). Systematic review: the epidemiology and natural history of non-alcoholic fatty liver disease and non-alcoholic steatohepatitis in adults. *Alimentary Pharmacology & Therapeutics*, **34**(3), 274–285.

16. Delormier, T., Frohlich, K.L., & Potvin, L. (2009). Food and eating as social practice – understanding eating patterns as social phenomena and implications for public health. *Sociology of Health & Illness*, **31**(2), 215–228.

17. Halkier, B., & Jensen, I. (2011). Doing 'healthier' food in everyday life? A qualitative study of how Pakistani Danes handle nutritional communication. *Critical Public Health*, **21**(4), 471–483.

18. Hinder, S., & Greenhalgh, T. (2012). 'This does my head in'. Ethnographic study of self-management by people with diabetes. *BMC Health Services Research*, **12**(1), 83.

19. Lau, A.Y., Arguel, A., Dennis, S., Liaw, S.-T., & Coiera, E. (2015). 'Why didn't it work?' Lessons from a randomized controlled trial of a Web-based personally controlled health management system for adults with asthma. *Journal of Medical Internet Research*, **17**(12), e283.

20. Davis, F.D. (1989). Perceived usefulness, perceived ease of use, and user acceptance of information technology. *MIS Quarterly*, **13**(3), 319–340.

21. Wherton, J., Sugarhood, P., Procter, R., Rouncefield, M., Dewsbury, G., Hinder, S., & Greenhalgh, T. (2012). Designing assisted living technologies 'in the wild': preliminary experiences with cultural probe methodology. *BMC Medical Research Methodology*, **12**, 188.

22. Wherton, J., Sugarhood, P., Procter, R., Hinder, S., & Greenhalgh, T. (2015). Co-production in practice: how people with assisted living needs can help design and evolve technologies and services. *Implementation Science*, **10**(1), 75.

23. Coiera, E. (2015). *Guide to Health Informatics*, 3rd edn. Boca Raton, FL, CRC Press.

24. Cross, N. (2006). *Designerly Ways of Knowing*. London, Springer.

25. Greenhalgh, T., Swinglehurst, D., & Stones, R. (2014). Rethinking 'resistance' to big IT: a sociological study of why and when healthcare staff do not use nationally mandated information and communication technologies. *Health Services and Delivery Research*, **39**(2), 1–86.

26. Rodriguez, C., & Pozzebon, M. (2005). A paradoxical world: exploring the discursive construction of collaboration in a competitive institutional context. In: *APROS 11: Asia-Pacific Researchers in Organization Studies: 11th International Colloquium, Melbourne, Australia, 4–7 December 2005: 2006 2005*, pp. 306–320.

27. Elwyn, G., Scholl, I., Tietbohl, C., Mann, M., Edwards, A.G., Clay, C., et al. 'Many miles to go…': a systematic review of the implementation of patient decision support interventions into routine clinical practice. *BMC Medical Informatics and Decision Making* 2013, **13**(2), 1.

28. Cherns, A. (1987). Principles of sociotechnical design revisted. *Human Relations*, **40**(3), 153–161.

29. Cherns, A. (1976). The principles of sociotechnical design. *Human Relations*, **29**(8), 783–792.

30. Clegg, C.W. (2000). Sociotechnical principles for system design. *Applied Ergonomics*, **31**(5), 463–477.

31. Markus, M.L. (1983). Power, politics, and MIS implementation. *Communications of the ACM*, **26**(6), 430–444.

32. Doolin, B. (2004). Power and resistance in the implementation of a medical management information system. *Information Systems Journal*, **14**(4), 343–362.

33. Carayon, P. (2006). Human factors of complex sociotechnical systems. *Applied Ergonomics*, **37**(4), 525–535.

34. Carayon, P., Wetterneck, T.B., Rivera-Rodriguez, A.J., Hundt, A.S., Hoonakker, P., Holden, R., & Gurses, A.P. (2014). Human factors systems approach to healthcare quality and patient safety. *Applied Ergonomics*, **45**(1), 14–25.

35. Symon, G., Long, K., & Ellis, J. (1996). The coordination of work activities: cooperation and conflict in a hospital context. *Computer Supported Cooperative Work*, **5**, 1–31.

36. Goorman, E., & Berg, M. (2000). Modelling nursing activities: electronic patient records and their discontents. *Nursing Inquiry*, **7**(1), 3–9.

37. Pratt, W., Reddy, M.C., McDonald, D.W., Tarczy-Hornoch, P., & Gennari, J.H. (2004). Incorporating ideas from computer-supported cooperative work. *Journal of Biomedical Informatics*, **37**(2), 128–137.

38. Greenhalgh, T., & Swinglehurst, D. (2011). Studying technology use as social practice: the untapped potential of ethnography. *BMC Medicine*, **9**, 45.

39. Han, Y.Y., Carcillo, J.A., Venkataraman, S.T., Clark, R.S., Watson, R.S., Nguyen, T.C., et al. (2005). Unexpected increased mortality after implementation of a commercially sold computerized physician order entry system. *Pediatrics*, **116**(6), 1506–1512.

40. Swinglehurst, D., Greenhalgh, T., & Roberts, C. (2012). Computer templates in chronic disease management: ethnographic case study in general practice. *BMJ Open*, **2**(6), pii.

41. Swinglehurst, D., Greenhalgh, T., Russell, J., & Myall, M. (2011). Receptionist input to quality and safety in repeat prescribing in UK general practice: ethnographic case study. *BMJ*, **343**, d6788.

42. Greenhalgh, T., & Stones, R. (2010). Theorising big IT programmes in healthcare: strong structuration theory meets actor-network theory. *Social Science & Medicine*, **70**, 1285–1294.

43. Greenhalgh, T., Stones, R., & Swinglehurst, D. (2014). Choose and book: a sociological analysis of 'resistance' to an expert system. *Social Science & Medicine*, **104**, 210–219.

Chapter 8

44. Sackett, D.L., Haynes, R.B., & Tugwell, P. (1985). *Clinical Epidemiology: A Basic Science for Clinical Medicine*. London, Little, Brown and Company.
45. Dourish, P., & Bell, G. (2011). *Divining a Digital Future: Mess and Mythology in Ubiquitous Computing*. Cambridge, MA, MIT Press.
46. Greenhalgh, T., Stramer, K., Bratan, T., Byrne, E., Russell, J., & Potts, H.W. (2010). Adoption and non-adoption of a shared electronic summary record in England: a mixed-method case study. *BMJ*, **340**, c3111.

Chapter 9 **Policy**

9.1 Evidence-based policy: beyond 'barriers and facilitators'

What do I mean by 'policy'? In the context of this book, I mean decisions that get made at national or local level about what health services will be funded and about how (and by whom) they will be delivered. Some examples of policy questions are given in Box 9.1.

The 'pipeline' model of research into practice (Section 2.2) suggests that the way to answer these questions is to commission research (new empirical studies and systematic reviews) into what works and then make a rational decision based on this research evidence. Much research into policymaking in healthcare begins with the assumption that evidence should be the starting point for policymaking, and that if we could identify 'barriers' (what stops policymakers using evidence) and 'facilitators' (what would help them), we could tweak the system to ensure that policy became unproblematically evidence-based.

Barriers-and-facilitators research on the policymaking process is so common that I have examined at least 10 PhDs whose output was yet another refinement of what is now a well-rehearsed taxonomy. All these candidates passed – but the policymaking process in their various localities and countries still is not evidence-based in the way the candidates had hoped, for reasons I will explain in the next section [1]. I am sure that more progress towards evidence-based policy would be made if, instead of doing evidence-focused studies of the research-into-policy pipeline, we instead did policy-focused research to *illuminate the complexity of how policymaking actually happens*. I review such research in Section 9.2, but first, let me give you a quick summary of some of the better barriers-and-facilitators studies in the literature.

How to Implement Evidence-Based Healthcare, First Edition. Trisha Greenhalgh.
© 2018 John Wiley & Sons Ltd. Published 2018 by John Wiley & Sons Ltd.

> **Box 9.1 Examples of policy questions**
> - Should we immunise teenage girls – and boys – against human papilloma virus?
> - Should breast reduction or enlargement ever be funded from the public purse?
> - To prevent type 2 diabetes, is it better to target lifestyle interventions (diet, exercise) to high-risk individuals, use population-wide approaches (e.g. tax sugary drinks, increase green spaces), or both?
> - At what age(s) (if at all) should babies and young children have developmental checks – and what should be checked at particular ages? Should these checks be done by specialist paediatricians, general practitioners, practice nurses or healthcare assistants?
> - What services should we offer in the community to reduce the number of frail older people who get re-admitted to hospital shortly after being discharged?
> - What should be our priorities when trying to reduce health inequalities?

One of the first such studies was done in 2000 by Heather Elliott and Jenny Popay, who demonstrated through qualitative interviews that the three main barriers to the use of evidence in policymaking were:

1. financial considerations (was the option affordable?);
2. shifting timescales (the evidence was not available when the policy decision needed to be made);
3. policymakers' own experiential knowledge (e.g. knowledge of what was going on locally, including what was already working) [2].

Elliot and Popay's interviews also showed that whilst it was relatively rare for research findings to have a direct influence on policy, research very often had an *indirect* influence – for example, by promoting public debate or shifting how some policymakers framed the issues (an important finding, which I will pick up in the next section).

Soon afterwards, a systematic review of the literature was published that listed three main 'facilitators' of use of evidence by policymakers:

1. personal contact with researchers,
2. timely relevance;
3. inclusion of summaries with policy recommendations [3].

This review also identified a number of barriers to the use of evidence by policymakers that had recurred in the empirical literature:

1. absence of personal contact with researchers;
2. lack of timeliness or relevance of the research;

3. mutual mistrust (the 'two cultures' problem – that academics and policymakers come from different worlds and find one another's priorities difficult to understand [4]);
4. power and budget struggles.

The same team updated its systematic review in 2014, and concluded:

> *The most frequently reported barriers to evidence uptake were poor access to good quality relevant research, and lack of timely research output. The most frequently reported facilitators were collaboration between researchers and policymakers, and improved relationships and skills.* [5]

If, like me, you do research for a living, you should reflect long and hard on the finding that in general, policymakers find the fruits of our labours difficult or impossible to use in practice. John Ioannidis' incisive paper, 'Why Most Clinical Research Is Not Useful', summarises the main reasons why this is the case [6]. The features listed in Box 2.1 are crucial to the practical relevance of a piece of research for both clinicians and policy-makers – yet few researchers ask all six questions before embarking on a study. As a result, all too often we produce a study that is (at best) metho-dologically robust but irrelevant to the questions being debated around the policymaking table.

Policymakers are not only interested in 'What works?' questions. As well as whether an intervention works, they also need to know – in clear and unambiguous terms – how much it will cost, how easy or difficult it will be to implement, whether it will have a knock-on effect on anything else (such as equity), whether the intervention tested was the best or the only option in the toolkit for that particular condition – and whether this issue is a priority compared to the dozens of other issues that are vying for attention at this point in time [1,7–9].

If you are keen to avoid adding to the mountain of policy-useless research, I encourage you to get hold of Christopher Whitty's masterly essay, 'What Makes an Academic Paper Useful for Policymakers?' (in which few of us in the research world get off scot-free) [8]. In sum, we academics tend to be too narrow in the questions we ask, too interested in randomised trials, not interested enough in questions of cost and cost-effectiveness, reluctant to synthesise evidence across a broad range of questions and methodologies, and incapable of writing plain-language summaries. To top it all, we usually take so long generating and polishing up our evidence that by the time it is available, the policy moment is past.

Chapter 9

In Whitty's words:

> *Academics underestimate the speed of the policy process, and publish excellent papers after a policy decision rather than good ones before it. To be useful in policy, papers must be at least as rigorous about reporting their methods as for other academic uses. Papers which are as simple as possible (but no simpler) are most likely to be taken up in policy. Most policy questions have many scientific questions, from different disciplines, within them. The accurate synthesis of existing information is the most important single offering by academics to the policy process. Since policymakers are making economic decisions, economic analysis is central, as are the qualitative social sciences. Models should, wherever possible, allow policymakers to vary assumptions. Objective, rigorous, original studies from multiple disciplines relevant to a policy question need to be synthesized before being incorporated into policy.* [8]

In sum, policymaking is a complex process, and one of the main reasons why policymakers do not fall over themselves looking for research evidence is that research is (traditionally) a self-serving industry that gives scant thought to what policymakers actually need. Although this has long been a problem, I do believe that things are getting better, as the later sections in this chapter argue.

9.2 How does policymaking actually happen?

Whilst the barriers-and-facilitators literature is useful up to a point, I set more store by ethnographic studies that seek to illuminate the complexities of policymaking in action. Such studies find that a huge range of evidence gets used in the policymaking process – not just research evidence, but also routinely collected data, financial modelling, expert opinion, the tacit knowledge and accumulated wisdom of frontline clinicians and public health practitioners, testimony from patients and citizens and so on [3,10,11]. Furthermore, as Elliot and Popay found back in 2000 (see Section 9.1), this evidence gets used in many different ways, both directly (to inform decisions) and indirectly (e.g. to inform debate or shift the way people view the problem).

One classic study in this genre is Carol Weiss' 1979 paper, 'The many meanings of research utilization' [12]. Weiss reviewed evidence from the social sciences on the impact of research on policy, and described four different modes of such impact. The first mode was *knowledge-driven* impact, in which fundamental discoveries are impelled into practice by their sheer innovative force. This, concluded Weiss, is extremely rare (for reasons that are now well-documented, and set out in Section 9.1). In short, the fantasy (common amongst naive researchers) of policymakers sitting around reading the *Lancet* and saying, 'Gosh, look at this research study, let's implement it right away' is, with very few exceptions, how policymaking *doesn't* happen!

Weiss's second mode of research impact was the *problem-solving* mode. Here, research is explicitly commissioned to solve particular policy problems, as in the infamous failed Rothschild experiment, in which the United Kingdom temporarily handed research budgets to policymakers, who were invited to act as 'customers' for academic research. Such an infrastructure (the ultimate set-up for evidence-based policymaking, some would argue) was established in the United Kingdom in 1972 – but had been disbanded by 1978. As Maurice Kogan and Mary Henkel showed in a gripping ethnographic study of how this all played out, despite political backing and resources, interactions between policymakers and scientists were awkward and largely unproductive; priority research topics were not readily identified; the (long) research commissioning cycle failed to align with the (short) policy cycle; and the quality and value of research was frequently questioned [13].

For these reasons, Rothschild's 1970s dream of systematically commissioned scientific research efficiently solving policy problems was never realised. As Weiss pointed out soon after Rothschild's customer-contractor model was junked, another reason why the problem-solving mode of research impact is rare is that scientific findings (especially in applied health research and the social sciences) tend to illuminate the complexity and contingency of phenomena, rather than providing simple and universal solutions to them [12].

Weiss's third mode of research impact was *interactional* – or, to use a more colloquial term, 'muddling through'. In other words, researchers and policymakers, through repeated interaction over time, come to understand one another's worlds and develop shared goals and approaches – Alexander George's famous 'two cultures' [4], traditionally at loggerheads, develop mutual awareness and even mutual respect.

As these researcher–policymaker interactions happen, research comes to influence the policy process, largely through non-linear mechanisms, including 'enlightenment' (as Steve Hanney's team puts it, 'the gradual "sedimentation" of insight, theories, concepts and perspectives' [14]) as a result of continuing exposure to research insights and ideas. Conversely, through the same interactions, researchers gradually wake up to the kind of research that policymakers might find useful and change the questions they ask and the methods they use.

The final mode of research impact in Weiss's taxonomy is *instrumental* (or *symbolic*) – a policymaker arms him- or herself with a particular piece of evidence in order to bolster a course of action he or she was intending to take anyway, or perhaps in order to delay a decision (arguing, perhaps, that new research must be commissioned in order to buy political breathing space) [12,14].

This last mode of how policymakers use research evidence might seem unscientific to the point of being manipulative, but let's remember that policy-making is as much about *values* as it is about objective science. Two recent papers have illustrated how systematic reviews are increasingly used by policymakers (and those seeking to lobby policymakers) [11,15]. Whilst it would be tempting to conclude that we have finally achieved a reliable evidence-into-policy pipeline, Smith and Stewart suggest that the utility of systematic reviews 'lies primarily in their symbolic value as markers of good decision making' [11].

One of the most important things to understand about the policymaking process is how some issues come to be seen as priorities at particular times and in particular contexts. John Kingdon's famous model of policy streams proposes that *potential* policies (or 'solutions') float around in a 'primordial soup' along with dynamically changing problems and the prevailing politics (Figure 9.1) [16]. How a definitive policy comes to bubble up from this primordial soup is beyond the scope of this book, but a lot depends on the presence of lobbyists and the rhetorical power with which they put their case.

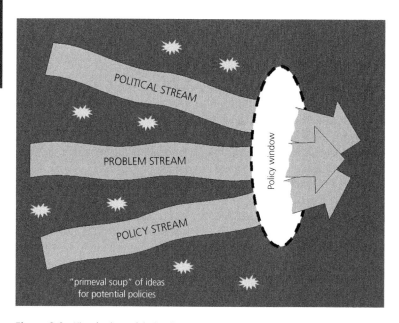

Figure 9.1 Kingdon's model of policy streams (based on [16]).

I once wrote a paper with Jill Russell, entitled 'Reframing evidence synthesis as rhetorical action in the policy making drama', in which we argued that policymaking is not a science but a science-informed practice, akin to social drama:

> *Policy making – which might be defined as the authoritative exposition of values – is about defining and pursuing the right course of action in a particular context, at a particular time, for a particular group of people and with a particular allocation of resources. Policy making is about making and implementing collective ethical judgements.* [10]

In a follow-up paper, we looked at the art of rhetoric and how it is used by those seeking to influence the policy process in order to persuade others of the legitimacy of their position [17]. Too often, policymaking is depicted as (purely) a rational exercise in decision science, in which the potential benefit of an intervention (e.g. an effect size from a randomised trial) is weighed against with the potential harm of that intervention *and* any challenges to the practicality or acceptability of the intervention *and* any competing calls on the funding pot. But there is a more fundamental process going on, too: policymakers need to *agree on what the questions are* in the first place – and on which questions should take priority. In other words, they need to *frame* the policy issue.

Let me illustrate what I mean by 'framing'. Drawing on the work of Judith Green [18], Jill Russell and I used the example of hip protectors – which at the time of writing had been shown in a systematic review of randomised trials to significantly reduce hip fracture in older people in residential homes [10]. In the 2000s, it briefly became fashionable to encourage residents to wear these devices (the 'evidence-based policy' of hip protectors in fracture prevention). But both staff and residents usually considered these products impractical and undignified (and, in an interesting battle of language, referred to them as 'padded knickers', not 'hip protectors').

Judith Green's initial analysis of this example centred on the competing framings of the problem. Was the issue 'risk of hip fractures' (from which older people needed to be protected) or was it 'dignity of residents' (and, in particular, their right to self-determination)? It was both, of course, and the fact that hip protectors never became standard policy in residential homes was due partly to the success of the 'dignity' framing, combined with the somewhat unconvincing nature of the evidence. Even on the evidence available in 2006, you would have had to put a lot of people through padded-knickers indignity for several years to prevent one fracture. In fact, a more recent systematic review found that hip protectors had no overall impact on the incidence of hip fracture [19].

Chapter 9

The policy questions in Box 9.1 can all be framed in more than one way. I recall that when immunisation of 13-year-old girls against human papilloma virus (HPV) was first introduced in the United Kingdom in 2007, some people framed it as 'preventing cervical cancer' whilst others framed it as 'encouraging promiscuity'. A few of my patients refused to allow their daughters to receive the vaccine at school in case anyone in their cultural community interpreted this as evidence that the girls were (or were planning to become) sexually active. They were in a minority, but had this been the majority position amongst parents, the policy would have fallen flat by failing the acceptability test.

Incidentally, the policy question of whether to immunise teenage *boys* against HPV has additional twists: Why should I expose my sons to a vaccine that is not going to protect *them* against cancer? The answer lies in the development of herd immunity. But economic analyses suggest that it is only cost-effective to immunise boys against HPV if the uptake amongst girls is low (otherwise, immunising the girls is all that is needed) [20]. All this and more will need to be taken into account when making local policy decisions on who to immunise against HPV (and whether to offer immunisation en masse at school or in the privacy of a doctor's clinic).

Here is another example. Prevention of type 2 diabetes is topical and controversial in the United Kingdom right now. This condition is rising rapidly in prevalence, especially amongst the poor and in black and minority ethnic groups. It is caused, broadly speaking, by an imbalance in energy intake (what you eat) versus energy expenditure (how much you exercise). The risk of developing type 2 diabetes is lowered in people who successfully reduce their energy intake and increase their levels of physical activity. Competing framings centre around whether preventive interventions should take a 'high-risk' approach and target selected individuals (with dietary education and encouragement to exercise more) or a 'population-wide' approach (measures such as increasing green spaces, making leisure centres free to those on low incomes, removing fizzy drink machines from schools, taxing sugar and so on) [21].

Randomised trials of targeted individual interventions have shown these to be effective in the high-risk populations studied, although it is not easy to identify who is at risk, and those most in need of the interventions may be least likely to take up the offer [22]. Those in favour of the population-wide approach have argued that high-risk policies are a political choice that amount to victim-blaming; they ignore the social determinants of health and the obesogenic environments in which disadvantaged communities tend to live [23].

I hope you can see from these brief examples that even when there is robust and relevant research evidence – but especially when the evidence is ambiguous, contested, incomplete or out of date – there is much, much more to policymaking than simply collecting and actioning the findings of randomised trials and systematic reviews. Arguing about what the questions are, and how they should be framed, is absolutely central to the policymaking process. This is why values (next section) are key, and no amount of research evidence will take the politics out of policymaking.

9.3 Value-based healthcare – and how values shape evidence

There is a lot of talk about both 'value' and 'values' (which are not quite the same thing) these days. I am sympathetic to much of what has been published, but I want to look critically at this area of work, since it sometimes leans towards oversimplifying the issues.

My friend and colleague Sir Muir Gray (whose claims to fame include coming up with the term 'evidence-based medicine' many years ago, thereby making clinical epidemiology infinitely more appealing to frontline clinicians) has spent the last 15 years or so working on what he calls 'value-based healthcare' [24] along with his US colleague Al Mulley (who introduced the term 'delivery science' to refer to the study of how to deliver services efficiently and equitably to populations [25]). Their use of the term 'value' is explicitly economic, and based on an influential paper on value for money in healthcare published by Michael Porter in 2009 [26].

The principle of value-based healthcare is simple (and difficult to argue with): there is now a substantial evidence base on which healthcare interventions work well, which work less well and which cause net harm. Some tests, and some treatments, are what Muir (along with his colleagues in the NHS RightCare group, previously known as the Preventing Overdiagnosis Group) calls 'high value' – that is, they are both effective and cost-effective. Others are what he calls 'low value' – that is, they are ineffective, harmful and/or not cost-effective. It would make sense for both national and local policymakers, who have a moral duty to maximise health benefits from a limited pot of money, to promote and support high-value interventions and take steps to curtail low-value ones.

In order to monitor progress towards high-value (and away from low-value) healthcare, the first thing we need, suggest Muir Gray and Al Mulley, is comparative data on how different geographical regions (or different healthcare providers) are performing with respect to one another. Policymakers can study these maps and benchmark local performance against best practice and against the national average. As the opening quote of Public Health England's (Muir Gray-inspired) Atlas of Variation says, 'When the approach in one town is major surgery and in another, it's watchful waiting, you know there's a problem' [27].

The US branch of the value-based healthcare movement is explicitly wedded to the idea of competition: if performance data are made publicly available, the best-performing providers will become known and attract more business, hence standards will be driven up (or so the argument goes) [28]. In the United Kingdom, the competitive dimension of value-based healthcare tends to be played down and the approach is framed more in terms of organisational learning and quality improvement.

Figure 9.2(a) shows one of the maps in the Atlas of Variation for England and Wales, whilst Figure 9.2(b) shows the same data in a histogram, with the apparently best-performing Clinical Commissioning Group (CCG) on the far left of the picture and the apparently worst-performing one on the far right. There is a fourfold difference between them. In all, the atlas contains 75 such maps, each of which illustrates a different indicator for which there is (said to be) good evidence that CCGs should be performing more consistently than is the case.

To talk you through an example, the rationale behind the inclusion of the indicator shown in Figure 9.2 is as follows. Almost four-fifths of antibiotic prescribing in the United Kingdom occurs in primary care, over half of which is for respiratory-tract infections. The level of such prescribing is increasing, and overprescribing relative to need is suspected to be one reason for this increase. The proportion of antibiotics from the cephalosporin, fluoroquinolone and co-amoxiclav classes (referred to in the Atlas as the 'key antibiotics' (as in 'key performance indicators', I guess)) is one of the UK Department of Health's Antimicrobial Prescribing Quality Measures (APQMs), because antibiotics from these classes are widely considered to be second-line treatment options for community-acquired infections [27]. Indiscriminate use of these drugs in primary care substantially increases the risk of antibiotic-induced infections such as *Clostridium difficile*. Each of the 75 variation maps includes a similar rationale based on a summary of research evidence.

The authors of the Atlas of Variation are careful *not* to state that the data as presented indicate that the CCGs shown darkest in the variation maps are the worst-performing – which is why I used the word 'apparently' in the paragraph before last. There are, of course, numerous possible explanations for me prescribing a cephalosporin in general practice (such as getting a letter from a specialist exhorting me to do just that for the patient whose care we share). Different geographical areas have different demographics and case mixes. CCGs at the extremes of performance may be highly atypical in this regard. So a map or graph of *variation* in the chosen indicator does not equate to a map or graph of good versus poor performance. But wide variation in something as important as the proportion of (ecologically dangerous) second-line antibiotics prescribed in general practice does cry out for an explanation.

The recommended response to apparent poor performance is shown in Figure 9.3. The map and graph shown in Figure 9.2 are the first phase of inquiry and are referred to as 'indicative' data, not 'evidential' data. The second phase is what the NHS RightCare group calls a 'deep-dive service review', along with

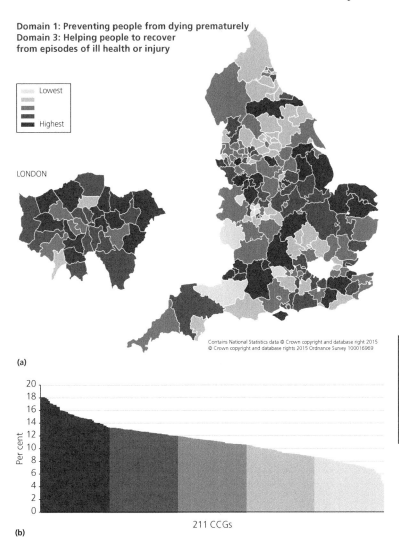

Domain 1: Preventing people from dying prematurely
Domain 3: Helping people to recover
from episodes of ill health or injury

Lowest

Highest

LONDON

Contains National Statistics data © Crown copyright and database right 2015
© Crown copyright and database rights 2015 Ordnance Survey 100016969

(a)

211 CCGs

(b)

Figure 9.2 (a) Example map from Public Health England's Atlas of Variation, showing the variation in the percentage of general practice antibiotic prescriptions that were for 'key' (i.e. second-line) antibiotics in England and Wales, 2015. (b) Example graph from Public Health England's Atlas of Variation: a histogram of 211 CCGs in England and Wales, 2015, showing a fourfold difference in the percentage of general practice antibiotic prescriptions that were for 'key' (second-line) antibiotics. *Source for both (a) and (b):* Public Health England [27]. © Crown copyright 2015. Licensed under the terms of the Open Government Licence v3.0.

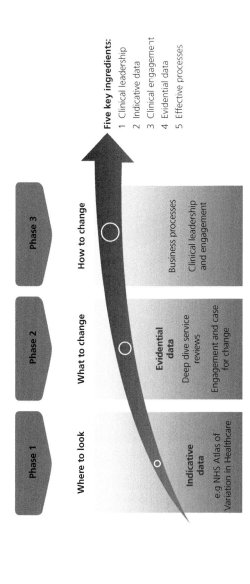

Figure 9.3 The NHS RightCare approach. *Source:* Public Health England [27]. © Crown copyright 2015. Licensed under the terms of the Open Government Licence v3.0.

clinical engagement (in other words, get the local doctors, nurses and pharmacists on board and gather plenty of detail on what's going on and why), aimed at producing, where appropriate, a case for change. The third phase is driving through change via the judicious application of the tools and techniques described in Appendix A (and beyond).

Many of the maps in the Atlas of Variation relate directly or indirectly to the kinds of policy decision made by the commissioners of local health services. For example, there are maps of variation in the proportion of cancers diagnosed at stage 4 (late), with the implication, perhaps, that the worst-performing areas might like to put more investment into screening. Maps of variation in the proportion of people transferred to a specialist stroke unit within 4 hours of admission for stroke suggest that the worst performers may wish to consider commissioning better stroke services. And so on.

All this seems very rational and sensible, and I'm sure much good would result if (i) everyone used such tools the way they were intended to be used; (ii) the tools were universally accepted as evidence-based indicators of variation that warrants investigation, not as league tables of good versus poor performers; (iii) data from variation maps, supplemented by 'deep-dive service reviews', could feed unproblematically into commissioning negotiations; and (iv) all or most of the challenges facing healthcare commissioners were amenable to the rational solutions that could be leveraged using the kind of data shown in Figure 9.1.

In reality, as inevitably happens when performance data are placed in the public domain, the data are sometimes misinterpreted and misused. 'Low value', which is shorthand for 'this intervention is *generally* not effective/cost-effective for target condition X', sometimes comes to be used as a blanket term to disparage the clinical decision in a *particular* case.

Even when policymakers aspire to be evidence-based and oriented to maximising value, they are not immune to the powerful framing effects of language. The reason I mentioned breast reduction and enhancement in Box 9.1 is that it topped the list of procedures that were considered in the work of 'rationing' panels in the UK National Health Service (NHS) [29]. These panels were established to adjudicate over appeals when a patient was turned down for NHS treatment on the grounds that the requested intervention was either ineffective or not cost-effective. In a research study a few years ago, my colleagues and I tape-recorded the deliberations of such panels about real cases (whose anonymised details were included in the paper with full patient consent). They included women whose breasts were so heavy that they had caused serious back pain and a 15-year-old boy who had grown a breast on one side and was deeply traumatised by teasing in the school locker room.

Almost all the requests for breast surgery that we observed fulfilled the criteria set out in the Royal College of Surgeons' commissioning guide on breast reduction surgery – which describes this procedure as a 'high-value treatment' [30]. Yet in every case, the appeal was rejected on the grounds that the operation counted as 'cosmetic surgery'. As we said in the paper, using the language of 'cosmetic surgery' (and even 'cosmetic boob jobs' – a term actually used in panel discussion) served a rhetorical purpose in these panels   to trivialise the medical condition and depict the patient, usually incorrectly, as motivated by vanity.

Breast reduction surgery is a good example of why an Atlas of Variation map might miss crucial detail. Plenty of women *do* seek breast reduction for cosmetic reasons (and in my view, that is a perfectly reasonable indication for the procedure so long as they pay for it themselves). But this means that comparing rates of breast reduction surgery across regions is not necessarily going to identify either under- or overperformance against the evidence-based guidelines.

The Atlas of Variation makes interesting reading, but the policymaking process for any condition – and commissioning decisions, in particular – is far more complex and involves far more variables than could ever be captured in a single performance indicator. To illustrate this, let us return to the example of the prevention of type 2 diabetes, which I began to explore in Section 9.2. It would be technically possible to produce small-area maps showing the proportion of people at high risk of developing type 2 diabetes who had been referred to a diabetes prevention programme (something Muir Gray, if he is up to date with his National Institute for Health and Care Excellence (NICE) guidelines, might reasonably classify as a 'high-value' intervention [31]). Using this logic, the 'high performers' would be the localities where individually-focused prevention programmes were thriving.

But such metrics would not address the wider policy question (about which there has rightly been much public deliberation recently): Should the government be putting the entire diabetes prevention budget into individually-focused preventive education rather than tackling obesogenic environments (and in particular, grasping the political nettle and taking on the junk food industry)? As I write this chapter (mid 2016), the UK government has just been criticised for a 'vacuous, vague and voluntary' national obesity policy of which an earlier draft had included compulsory restrictions on the marketing of energy-dense, nutrient-poor foods to children. The Prime Minister was said to have over-ruled the Secretary of State for Health on the grounds that the economic benefits to the food industry of *not* having such restrictions were of higher political importance than the health benefits to citizens of having them [32].

Whichever way you swing on the question of whether type 2 diabetes and the obesity that predisposes to it are the result of individual choice or environmental pressures, I hope this example will serve my purpose to show that 'facts', even when derived from high-quality randomised trials or observational studies, are inevitably value-laden. As Mike Kelly and colleagues argued recently, values (i.e. the things we hold to be important and morally good) influence every aspect of the evidence-based healthcare (EBHC) process [33], from the choice of topics that should be researched to the particular questions asked by researchers, the study designs deemed valid, the way results are interpreted and presented, and which conclusions are drawn.

If, for example, the funders of research place high value on the remediable social determinants of health (such as poverty, low health literacy, discrimination, inadequate housing and so on), they will be more likely to put money into mixed-method research to explore the nature of health inequalities, natural experiments of community-based interventions and the impact of fiscal measures such as sugar tax and restrictions on advertising. If, on the other hand, funders place high value on individual responsibility for lifestyle 'choices', they will be more likely to allocate funding to randomised trials of dietary education and prescription-for-exercise schemes. And if the lion's share of research evidence consists of the latter kinds of study, we should expect the resulting NICE guidelines on diabetes prevention to focus predominantly on interventions delivered to individuals.

To return to value-based health care, I am all for careful measurement of geographical variation in practice and the use of such data to prompt reflection on what is causing such variation. But I believe that because the 'facts' generated by such tools are value-laden, we should always ask critical questions about why particular indicators have been selected, what alternative explanations are possible for the findings presented and – most importantly of all, perhaps – which dimensions of illness and aspects of care are not being measured and why.

9.4 Ten tips for closer alignment between research and policy

1. Recognise the wide range of evidence that gets used by policymakers

In Section 9.1, I gave examples of the diversity of evidence sources that policymakers find useful. Indeed, it would be impossible for policymakers to do their jobs without (for example) routinely collected data about burden of disease, uptake and use of local services, the accumulated wisdom of local experts (of various kinds), testimony from local clinicians and patients, the perspective of advocates and lobbyists, and such things as press reports on what issues are viewed as local priorities. Your contribution of research evidence will not sit above these other sources on a silver platter. Rather, it will need to earn its place in a patchwork of all these evidence sources. It will be more likely to fit seamlessly with the full body of evidence if it addresses the issues and contextual factors identified in all the other evidence sources [9].

2. Get your head round why most research is not useful to policymakers

Section 9.1 provides a summary of why so much research that is undertaken with the intention of informing policy does not actually prove useful. The policy cycle is fast-paced and punctuated with fixed deadlines. It needs broad-based, interdisciplinary evidence with a clear bottom line, including evidence of likely impacts and costs. This fits poorly with the current fetish for randomised trials that produce precise answers to very narrow questions and make little effort to estimate likely real-world costs.

3. Learn and apply some health economics

Right from the very earliest studies on the use (and non-use) of research evidence by policymakers, findings have consistently shown that a major barrier is mismatch between the recommendations from research and the funds available to implement those recommendations (see Section 9.1). Policymakers want to know not just what the most effective interventions cost but also whether there is a next-best option that is a little less effective but significantly cheaper. In *How to Read a Paper*, I included a chapter on 'Papers that Tell You What Things Cost', which explained some of the research designs that produce cost-effectiveness data [34]. Healthcare policymakers are very keen on modelling studies – in which different assumptions and what-if scenarios are compared and the cost implications are estimated. Economic modelling is not my field of expertise, but a couple of papers by Mark Schulpher and Pelham Barton will get you started [35,36].

4. Consider the four ways in which research evidence is actually used by policymakers

In Section 9.2, I introduced the work of Carol Weiss, who considered four modes of evidence use by policymakers, and the likelihood of spotting each mode in practice:

- knowledge-driven mode – almost never;
- problem-solving mode – extremely rare;
- interactional mode – common;
- instrumental mode – ubiquitous.

This, of course, means that you need to interact with policymakers (see Tip 5) and anticipate that the evidence you produce is quite likely to be used instrumentally in the contact sport of frontline policymaking.

5. Build relationships with policymakers

As I mentioned in Section 9.1, personal relationships between the people who do research and the people who (we would like to) use research are important facilitators of research utilisation by policymakers. Do not wait until you have research data to show a policymaker – make friends with him or her before you even apply for your grant! I have lost count of the number of briefing breakfasts I have attended, organised by the Nuffield Trust, the King's Fund and similar knowledge-brokering organisations ('think tanks'). Such events are far from a waste of time, so seek them out and build them into your timetable. The next chapter, on networks and networking, may give you some more concrete ideas on how to go about this.

6. Produce policy-relevant summaries of evidence

Remember the quote given in Section 9.1: 'The accurate synthesis of existing information [from different disciplines] is the most important single offering by academics to the policy process' [8]. With this in mind, pick a topic and embark on a scoping review. But note also Whitty's advice to stop short of telling policymakers their job:

> *Don't feel the need to spell out policy implications. This may sound counter-intuitive, but many good scientific papers are let down by simplistic, grandiose or silly policy implications sections. Policymaking is a professional skill; most scientists have no experience of it and it shows.* [8]

7. Be aware of the power of framing – and develop frame awareness

As described in Section 9.2, much of policymaking is argument about the best course of action. A key to achieving this effectively is the development of a critical awareness of the rhetorical use of language, by both oneself and others – a state that Rein and Schön have called 'frame-reflective awareness' [37]. Awareness of our frames (i.e. the conceptual and perceptual lenses through which we view the world) can help expose the different systems of values, preferences and beliefs in which we and our opponents are arguing. Such awareness will also illuminate how we (and they) construct and position potential audiences – and more fundamentally, how we formulate and construct what 'the problem' is in the first place. A good way to get started on this task is to look for opposing views on a policy topic and pull out how problems and solutions are presented in each perspective.

Chapter 9

8. Value data – but remember that all data are value-laden

See Tip 1. Policymakers need reliable and timely data on what is going on locally and nationally – and in particular, the extent to which current perform ance is in line with the best available evidence. In Section 9.3, I used the Atlas of Variation as an example of the kind of data that can be used to bench-mark performance and attempt to improve the ratio of high- to low-value care that is delivered. But I also cautioned against seeing such data as capable of providing the full picture of what services are needed in a locality or a precise hierarchy of which interventions are the most worthwhile. Reality is much messier – and, as I argued earlier, the evidence may contain numerous hidden assumptions and value-judgements.

9. Work actively to bridge the 'two cultures' divide

As noted in Section 9.1, researchers and policymakers come from different worlds [4]. It takes a lot of effort and persistence to reach an understanding of a different culture. But such effort and persistence is likely to pay off in the long term. The final sentence in the final report of an evaluation I led of a long and complex national IT programme reads as follows:

> *Dialogue (or lack of it) occurs in the context of multiple conflicting worlds (political, clinical, technical, commercial, academic and personal – and probably others as well). Strong feelings, misunderstandings, conflicting values and competing priorities are to be expected – and we offer no magic recipe for resolving them. But we do offer an observation from three years' involvement with these complex programmes: greatest progress appeared to be made when key stakeholders came together in uneasy dialogue, speaking each other's languages imperfectly and trying to understand where others were coming from, even when the hoped-for consensus never materialised. [38]*

10. Seek to influence research policy

This chapter has been about health policy, and the ways in which people who make health policy use research (and other kinds of) evidence. There is another, related, kind of policy: the decisions that are made to prioritise topics for research, invite applications for funding, allocate funding to particular research projects and programmes, and promote links between healthcare researchers and those in other disciplines. Research policy, like health policy, is based on values and develops through argument and persuasion. If you want to influence how research money is allocated, apply to sit on the panels that allocate it. You will not get things all your own way, but you may be able to influence the research process to help make it more engaged with the needs of healthcare policymakers.

References

1. Greenhalgh, T., & Russell, J. (2009). Evidence-based policymaking: a critique. *Perspectives in Biology and Medicine*, **52**(2), 304–318.
2. Elliott, H., & Popay, J. (2000). How are policy makers using evidence? Models of research utilisation and local NHS policy making. *Journal of Epidemiology and Community Health*, **54**(6), 461–468.
3. Innvær, S., Vist, G., Trommald, M., & Oxman, A. (2002). Health policy-makers' perceptions of their use of evidence: a systematic review. *Journal of Health Services Research & Policy*, **7**(4), 239–244.
4. George, A.L. (1994). The two cultures of academia and policy-making: bridging the gap. *Political Psychology*, **15**(1), 143–172.
5. Oliver, K., Innvar, S., Lorenc, T., Woodman, J., & Thomas, J. (2014). A systematic review of barriers to and facilitators of the use of evidence by policymakers. *BMC Health Services Research*, **14**(1), 2.
6. Ioannidis, J.P. (2016). Why most clinical research is not useful. *PLoS Medicine*, **13**(6):e1002049.
7. Petticrew, M., Whitehead, M., Macintyre, S.J., Graham, H., & Egan, M. (2004). Evidence for public health policy on inequalities. 1: The reality according to policymakers. *Journal of Epidemiology and Community Health*, **58**(10), 811–816.
8. Whitty, C.J. (2015). What makes an academic paper useful for health policy? *BMC Medicine*, **13**(1), 1.
9. Moat, K.A., Lavis, J.N., & Abelson, J. (2013). How contexts and issues influence the use of policy-relevant research syntheses: a critical interpretive synthesis. *The Milbank Quarterly*, **91**(3), 604–648.
10. Greenhalgh, T., & Russell, J. (2006). Reframing evidence synthesis as rhetorical action in the policy making drama. *Healthcare Policy/Politiques de Santé*, **1**(2), 34–42.
11. Smith, K.E., & Stewart, E. (2015). 'Black magic' and 'gold dust': the epistemic and political uses of evidence tools in public health policy making. *Evidence & Policy*, **11**(3), 415–437.
12. Weiss, C.H. (1979). The many meanings of research utilization. *Public Administration Review*, **39**(5), 426–431.
13. Kogan, M., & Henkel, M. (1983). *Government and Research: The Rothschild Experiment in a Government Department*. London, Heinemann Educational Books.
14. Hanney, S.R., Gonzalez-Block, M.A., Buxton, M.J., & Kogan, M. (2003). The utilisation of health research in policy-making: concepts, examples and methods of assessment. *Health Research Policy and Systems*, **1**(1), 2.
15. Fox, D.M. (2011). Systematic reviews and health policy: the influence of a project on perinatal care since 1988. *The Milbank Quarterly*, **89**(3), 425–449.
16. Kingdon, J.W. (1984). *Agendas, Alternatives, and Public Policies*. Boston, MA, Little, Brown and Company.
17. Russell, J., Greenhalgh, T., Byrne, E., & McDonnell, J. (2008). Recognizing rhetoric in health care policy analysis. *Journal of Health Services Research & Policy*, **13**(1), 40–46.

Chapter 9

18. Green, J. (2000). Epistemology, evidence and experience: evidence based health care in the work of accident alliances. *Sociology of Health & Illness*, **22**(4), 453–476.

19. Parker, M.J., Gillespie, W.J., & Gillespie, L.D. (2006). Effectiveness of hip protectors for preventing hip fractures in elderly people: systematic review. *BMJ*, **332**(7541), 571–574.

20. Kim, J.J., & Goldie, S.J. (2009). Cost effectiveness analysis of including boys in a human papillomavirus vaccination programme in the United States. *BMJ*, **339**, b3884.

21. Rose, G. (2001). Sick individuals and sick populations. *International Journal of Epidemiology*, **30**(3), 427–432.

22. Barry, E., Roberts, S., Oke, J., Vijayaraghavan, S., Normansell, R., & Greenhalgh, T. (2016). Can type 2 diabetes be prevented using screen-and-treat policies? Systematic review and meta-analysis of screening tests and interventions for pre-diabetes. *BMJ*, submitted.

23. Barry, E., Roberts, S., Finer, S., Vijayaraghavan, S., & Greenhalgh, T. (2015). Time to question the NHS diabetes prevention programme. *BMJ*, **351**, h4717.

24. Gray, M., & El Turabi, A. (2012). Optimising the value of interventions for populations. *BMJ*, **345**, e6192.

25. Mulley, A.G. Jr. (2013). The global role of health care delivery science: learning from variation to build health systems that avoid waste and harm. *Journal of General Internal Medicine*, **28**(3), 646–653.

26. Porter, M.E. (2007). Clusters and Economic Policy: Aligning Public Policy with the New Economics of Competition. White Paper (Institute for Strategy and Competitiveness, Harvard Business School).

27. Public Health England (2015). Atlas of Variation. Available from: https://fingertips.phe.org.uk/profile/atlas-of-variation (last accessed 14 January 2017).

28. Harvard Business School Institute for Strategy and Competitiveness (2016). Value-Based Health Care Delivery. Available from: http://www.isc.hbs.edu/health-care/vbhcd/pages/default.aspx (last accessed 14 January 2017).

29. Russell, J., Swinglehurst, D., & Greenhalgh, T. (2014). 'Cosmetic boob jobs' or evidence-based breast surgery: an interpretive policy analysis of the rationing of 'low value' treatments in the English National Health Service. *BMC Health Services Research*, **14**(1), 413.

30. Royal College of Surgeons (2014). Breast Reduction – Commissioning Guide. Available from: http://www.rcseng.ac.uk/healthcare-bodies/docs/breast-reduction-commissioning-guide (last accessed 14 January 2017).

31. National Institute for Health and Clinical Excellence (2012). Type 2 Diabetes: Prevention in People at High Risk (NICE Guideline 38). Available from: https://www.nice.org.uk/guidance/ph38 (last accessed 14 January 2017).

32. Siddique, H., & Syal, R. (2016). Theresa May's First Test was Obesity and She has Failed, Say Health Experts. Available from: https://www.theguardian.com/society/2016/aug/21/theresa-mays-first-test-was-obesity-strategy-and-she-has-failed-health-experts-say (last accessed 14 January 2017).

33. Kelly, M.P., Heath, I., Howick, J., & Greenhalgh, T. (2015). The importance of values in evidence-based medicine. *BMC Medical Ethics*, **16**(1), 69.

34. Greenhalgh, T. (2014). *How to Read a Paper: The Basics of Evidence-Based Medicine.* Chichester, John Wiley & Sons.
35. Sculpher, M.J., Claxton, K., Drummond, M., & McCabe, C. (2006). Whither trial-based economic evaluation for health care decision making? *Health Economics,* **15**(7), 677–687.
36. Barton, P., Bryan, S., & Robinson, S. (2004). Modelling in the economic evaluation of health care: selecting the appropriate approach. *Journal of Health Services Research & Policy,* **9**(2), 110–118.
37. Rein, M., & Schön, D. (1993). Reframing policy discourse. In: F. Fischer and J. Forester (eds). *The Argumentative Turn in Policy Analysis and Planning.* Durham, NC, Duke University Press Books.
38. Greenhalgh, T., Stramer, K., Bratan, T., Byrne, E., Russell, J., Hinder, S., & Potts, H. (2010). *The Devil's in the Detail: Final Report of the Independent Evaluation of the Summary Care Record and HealthSpace Programmes.* London, University College London.

Chapter 9

Chapter 10 **Networks**

10.1 Networks and knowledge

Adapting a sentence originally penned by Penny Hawe and colleagues [1], I define a network as:

> *the relationships that exist between groups of individuals or agencies, the resources to which membership of such groups facilitates access and the opportunities for knowledge creation that arise from these relationships and resources.*

Networks (of many different kinds) are key to the generation and transfer of knowledge between people, teams, organisations and sectors [2]. This chapter is not a comprehensive account of every kind of network. Rather, it offers eclectic examples of networks that are important for the implementation of EBHC. Networks overlap considerably with systems. In the next chapter, I will cover the kinds of network that are best thought of as complex systems, including actor networks (i.e. networks of people and technologies as conceptualised by actor–network theory: Section 11.3) and multi-stakeholder health research systems (Section 11.4).

In Section 10.2, I give a brief account of social network theory as applied to both individuals and organisations. In Section 10.3, I cover professional communities of practice and introduce the concept of collectively constructed mindlines (which, arguably, influence evidence-based practice more than written guidelines). In Section 10.4, I consider the parallel phenomenon of lay networks – important sources of knowledge amongst patients and carers that are (in my view) researched too little and in an overly medicalised way. Finally, Section 10.5 offers some tips for creating better networks and doing better networking.

Key to understanding how all the networks covered in this chapter and the next contribute to the implementation of EBHC is a broader conceptualisation

How to Implement Evidence-Based Healthcare, First Edition. Trisha Greenhalgh.
© 2018 John Wiley & Sons Ltd. Published 2018 by John Wiley & Sons Ltd.

of what knowledge *is*. My advice: stop thinking of knowledge as atomistic facts that sit tidily in individual people's heads. Knowledge may occasionally be precisely that, but it is also something more: it is the understandings and framings that are *shared* amongst groups of individuals (or, at an even higher level, groups of organisations) [3,4]. Furthermore, knowledge is produced (i.e. generated and refined) *by* groups of people [5]. This is why networks and networking are so important.

Knowledge, as developed by and circulated amongst networks, is a fickle beast. It is sometimes explicit (the kind of knowledge you can write down, define precisely and send as an email attachment) and sometimes tacit (the embodied knowledge about, say, how to ride a bicycle, remove an appendix or raise a child – knowledge that, in short, cannot be precisely defined or reduced to a set of instructions) [6]. And it is often multiple – by which I mean, there is rarely consensus within the network.

Indeed, a network can be thought of as the linkages and interactions through which knowledge is agreed upon (rarely), negotiated (more commonly), valued or devalued (variously) and – above all – contested. Susan Leigh Star, who knew a thing or two about networks, once defined a discipline (i.e. a network of academics) as 'a commitment to engage in disagreements' [7]. And as Paulo Friere puts it, 'Knowledge emerges only through invention and reinvention, through the restless, impatient, continuing, hopeful inquiry men pursue in the world, with the world, and with each other' [8] (we might, these days, add 'and women').

This dynamic, contested and emergent view of knowledge is a good place to start when thinking about why networks are important to implementing EBHC. But surely, you may ask, the whole point of EBHC is finding out what is *the best* approach and then ensuring that this gets standardised everywhere, so what is there to argue about? It is true that networks are important for spreading knowledge even when there is no disagreement. But it is also true that, in real life (as opposed to the thought-experiments enjoyed by theorists), evidence needs to be weighed up, interpreted, assessed as more or less relevant, applied to the here and now of a particular local setting (e.g. the evidence-based guideline may recommend drug A but the hospital formulary offers only drug B) and considered in the light of competing priorities and concerns (see my discussion on framing in Section 9.2). Hence, there is often a need to argue it out.

Different perspectives on knowledge depend on different philosophical positions on the nature of reality. Contandriopoulos et al. [3] depicted knowledge in two essential forms (although with much dynamic overlap between them): individual – that is, held in people's heads and translated (or not) into action by human will and agency (a conception of knowledge that rests largely on positivist assumptions of a hard external reality); and

Chapter 10

collective – that is, socially shared and organisationally embedded (a conception that rests on more interpretivist philosophical assumptions). These authors reviewed the mechanisms by which knowledge may become collectivised, including efforts to make it relevant, legitimate and accessible and to take account of the values and priorities of a particular audience. If there is broad agreement on what the problem is and what a solution would look like, arguments about implementing evidence can proceed along the lines of conventional scientific inquiry (e.g. strength of research evidence). If not, the knowledge mobilisation challenge enters the more fluid and subjective realm of political science – in which research use is, in Carol Weiss's taxonomy (explained in Section 9.2), instrumental (tactical) rather than knowledge-driven [9].

These days, social media (Facebook, Twitter and the like) is key to the generation, circulation, interpretation and contestation of knowledge in both professional and lay networks. In an earlier draft of this chapter, I included social media as a separate section. But I found it made more sense to include such technologies as part of wider (human *and* technological) networks than to study them in isolation. For this reason, technology runs as a thread through all the sections of this chapter (and I suspect that particular thread will need regular updating).

10.2 Social network analysis

A social network has been defined as 'the pattern of friendship, advice, communication or support which exists among members of a social system' [10]. The principles of social network theory are summarised in Box 10.1.

Everett Rogers was a sociologist who developed diffusion of innovations theory back in the 1950s. His research group produced the attributes of innovations described in Section 2.4, and came up with the famous innovation adoption curve (Figure 10.1) in relation to the adoption of new farming practices in rural America [11]. This work included the important discovery that the more contacts a person has with other people in their social network, the more likely they are to be an innovator or an early adopter of an innovation (Figure 10.1) rather than a late adopter or 'laggard'. As Rogers himself emphasised, we have to be careful using such value-laden terms, which effectively imply that adopting any innovation is always good and that being a 'laggard' is always bad – whereas this is only actually the case if the innovation is beneficial rather than a passing fad (on which, more later).

Shortly after Rogers' team had published its initial work on the diffusion of new farming practices, James Coleman's team from Columbia University published near-identical findings (including another S-shaped adoption curve) amongst US doctors who were being encouraged to prescribe the

---

Box 10.1 Principles of social network theory

1 **Social relationships:** All behaviour is embedded in social relationships, hence the adoption and diffusion of innovations are driven by the social relationships amongst actors.

2 **Strength of weak ties:** The links in a social network are classified primarily according to the degree to which they convey new information. Individuals who are linked by weak social ties potentially have more information to share with one another.

3 **Structural equivalence:** The degree to which two individuals have the same relations with the same others. People with structural equivalence tend to adopt an innovation with a similar level of exposure.

4 **Threshold models:** We each have a threshold for adopting an innovation according to how many others have already done so. Early adopters are those whose threshold for adopting the innovation is low (they will do so when only a few people in the social system have already done so); late adopters will only adopt once most others in their social system have done so.

5 **Opinion leader:** An individual who has unusually high influence over the behaviour of others in his or her social network, by virtue of charisma, competence, connectedness and perceived homophily (i.e. similarity to the intended adopter).

Source: Summarised from various sources [10–13].

---

antibiotic tetracycline [14]. The study was funded by Pfizer, the manufacturer of the new drug, who wanted to learn the best marketing techniques to persuade doctors to prescribe their products.

When Coleman et al. observed the critical importance of personal contacts in influencing doctors' decision-making, they extended their study into an exploration of the doctors' social networks. This 'sociogram', as it was called – a mapping exercise of who knows whom and who influences whom, usually done on a computer these days – produced what Everett Rogers called 'one of the most important diffusion studies of all time'. Coleman's team obtained independent evidence of the time taken to first prescribe tetracycline using local pharmacists' dispensing records. It produced profiles of doctors identified by their colleagues as influencing their decision to prescribe – people we would now designate 'opinion leaders'. Coleman's team found that time to adoption of the new drug depended heavily on the size and quality of the doctors' social networks and on how often they went to out-of-town medical meetings.

The Coleman study was taken up by mainstream sociology as a paradigm for studying the social networks of potential adopters of innovations. It also

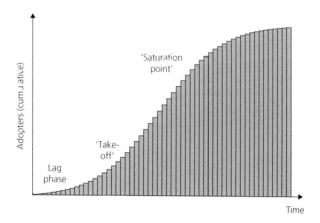

Figure 10.1   S-shaped adoption curve.

had a critical influence on the pharmaceutical industry's marketing strategies: from this study was born the pharmaceutical representative or 'detailer', the 'drug lunch' (pharmaceutical sponsorship of social gatherings of doctors) and efforts by pharmaceutical companies to identify and influence 'opinion leading' physicians – marketing tactics that persist (and remain ethically questionable [15]) to this day. The same findings also influenced the EBHC movement to introduce educational outreach by people independent of the pharmaceutical industry and mobilisation of local opinion leaders to counter the powerful influence of interpersonal marketing tactics [16,17].

Central to social network theory is the notion that the embeddedness of an individual in a social system (i.e. the number and extent of their relationships) is positively related to where they sit on the S-shaped innovation adoption curve [14,18]. The 'weak ties' concept (Box 10.1) introduced by Granovetter [12] is somewhat counter-intuitive, but it makes sense because individuals with strong interpersonal ties (spouses, best friends, people who work in the same office) already share large amounts of information, whereas those with weak ties (past acquaintances, friends of friends) have potentially more information to exchange. Hence, the best source of new ideas is often someone one hardly knows. The type and direction of social influence is different in different professional groups: one classic study showed that doctors tend to be influenced by peers ('cliques'), whereas nurses are more influenced by their seniors ('hierarchies') [19], although I doubt that these findings are universally transferable.

Since this early work, social network analysis has become a sophisticated (and, dare I say it, jargon-bound and methodologically intense) science that rests increasingly on statistical analysis. Whilst the basic principles and landmark studies described here are important, I am not a great fan of the more contemporary developments in the discipline. I find most studies data-heavy on who links with whom but data-light on what happens through these connections and why it matters. I guess I have examined too many PhDs in which the candidate spent years producing and validating a computer-generated sociogram but added little to the overall theory. But if social network analysis is what floats your boat, a paper from Penny Hawe's team is a great way to take your knowledge beyond the basics described in this section [1].

In my view, the most important thing for a non-expert to take from the literature on social network theory is that certain individuals have a great deal of influence on whether someone adopts an innovation (and, broadly speaking, this influence can be classified as positive if the innovation is evidence-based and negative if it is not). The main types of influencer are shown in Box 10.2.

One thing that is sometimes insufficiently stressed in the EBHC literature is that interpersonal influence is a *social process* that occurs in real-world settings. Whilst there have been dozens of randomised trials studying the influence of opinion leaders and other individuals on clinical behaviour, I am skeptical of their findings, which tend to suggest modest effects [17]. I think this is because social influence does not lend itself well to experimentation. For example, you cannot simply ship in an individual who has credibility

---

Box 10.2 Social influencers

- **Peer opinion-leaders:** We tend to copy people we see as being like us (what Rogers called 'homophily'). Some people, at the centre of their peer networks, have a lot of influence.
- **Expert opinion leaders:** People we see as more skilled or knowledgeable than us (e.g. senior consultants or professors). The relative influence of peer versus opinion leaders in different contexts is complex and almost certainly context-dependent.
- **Champions:** People who feel positively about a particular idea or practice and voluntarily seek to persuade others of its value. Whether a champion is effective in changing behaviour will depend to a large extent on whether he or she is also a peer or expert opinion leader.
- **Knowledge brokers (or knowledge intermediaries):** People who are employed with the explicit purpose of disseminating knowledge to particular target groups of people (most commonly, clinicians in an organisation). Whereas much of the influence of opinion leaders and champions is unintended, knowledge brokers set out with the explicit purpose of influencing others (indeed, that task will be high on their official job description).

Chapter 10

with the people walking the floor any more than you can experimentally manipulate the atmosphere at a party.

I am more impressed by the work of qualitative researchers who have undertaken ethnographic studies in the workplace and documented the subtle but profound influences that peer opinion leaders (sometimes) have. For example, in an old but classic paper, Louise Locock's team reports on a large study of the implementation of evidence across 22 healthcare organisations using an in-depth case-study design [20]. Locock et al.'s conclusion is worth quoting:

> *Three factors stood out as particularly influential [in the success or otherwise of the project]: the strength and clarity of the evidence which the project sought to implement; the committed support of key opinion leaders; and the extent of wider organisational commitment to evidence-based practice.*

A relatively recent development in the study of social networks is formal analysis of social media profiles. Coleman et al.'s use of 'attendance at out-of-town medical meetings' as a measure of social connectedness in the early 1960s now reads as decidedly quaint. These days, someone repeating Coleman's study would presumably have to assess the doctors' LinkedIn profiles, number of Twitter followers and participation in medical Facebook communities.

I am a keen user of Twitter myself (you can follow me on @trishgreenhalgh), and occasionally receive automated notices along the lines of, 'Congratulations, you are number 4 on our Top Medical Influencers list this week'. Presumably, the organisations sending these notices have somehow measured how many other people 'liked' or 'retweeted' a message I posted. I have to say, I do not take much notice of these alerts – but perhaps I should. Sociologist Deborah Lupton studies academic networks and has produced an excellent summary chapter on 'The Digitised Academic' for those interested in pursuing the topic further [21].

One final theme to introduce in this section is how the unit of analysis in a social network analysis can be the organisation instead of the individual. Back in 2004, my team's review of the literature on how innovations spread in healthcare included a whole chapter on inter-organisational networks [22]. Just as individuals copy other individuals (and more so if those individuals are homophilic and recognised as opinion leaders), so organisations follow other ('exemplar') organisations according to very similar principles. Organisations tend to copy other organisations of similar size, ethos, strategic mission, maturity and so on [22]. And just as some individuals are more embedded than others in their social networks, so are some organisations.

Amongst similar organisations, there is a good deal of inter-organisational norm-setting and benchmarking [22]. In other words, when the board of an organisation considers whether to take on an innovation (say, computerised prescribing), one of the first questions that will be asked is, 'Are they doing this at hospital X yet?' – where hospital X is the acknowledged leader in relation to information and communication technologies. The organisational parallels with social network theory are summarised in Box 10.3.

Exchange of ideas between organisations occurs best when individuals from those organisations can interact extensively (via such things as secondments, collaborative projects, job changes, conferences and networking events). Granovetter (of 'weak ties' fame) [12] argued that weak ties were particularly important for allowing innovations to spread across subgroups within a system because they provide access to novel information by creating bridges between otherwise disconnected individuals.

To some extent, inter-organisational linkage and benchmarking is extremely helpful for the spread of new practices in EBHC, since it means that once an opinion-leading organisation has come on board to an innovative practice or service model, other organisations will be asking themselves whether they should come on board too. But as Eric Abrahamson showed in his classic 1991 paper, this 'bandwagon phenomenon' also means that ideas and practices with no demonstrable benefit and even potential for harm

---

Box 10.3 Some organisational parallels from social network theory

1 **Organisational fads and fashions:** Innovations spread between organisations by copying.

2 **Organisational opinion leaders or 'exemplars':** Certain organisations come to be seen as leading-edge.

3 **Organisational ties:** The extent and direction of flows between, and closeness amongst, organisations. Ties can be indirect (mediated through a third party) or direct (which are expected to be stronger). The stronger the ties, the more innovative the organisation.

4 **Organisational centrality:** An organisation's position within a network, measured by resource and information flows and social ties (the greater the centrality of an organisation, the more innovative it might be expected to be).

5 **Redundancy:** Where two organisations provide a third with the same information.

6 **Structural holes:** Where two organisations are tied to a third but not to one another.

Source: [10–12,18,23].

Chapter 10

(what he called 'organisational fads and fashions') can spread quickly amongst like-minded organisations [23]. And, of course, such spread will be accelerated by the very inter-organisational networking events that are intended to spread best practice. If you want an example of how fads and fashions in healthcare strategy were spread far beyond their usefulness through a bandwagon effect, one is provided by Kaissi & Begun [24].

In sum, social networking both between individuals and (through them) between organisations can be a powerful force for good in the spread of best practice – but it can also spread *poor* practice. Social influence is, as the name implies, a social phenomenon, so (in my personal view) studies in which researchers have attempted to manipulate it like an experimental variable have tended to produce equivocal, questionable and somewhat uninteresting results.

10.3 Professional communities of practice and 'mindlines'

The previous section concerned social influence on the adoption of innovations (such as a new drug or service model). This section is about the influence of others on professional practice. Jean Lave is a social scientist who, with Etienne Wenger, developed the notion of *communities of practice*. In an early article, she exhorted those who study knowledge and its acquisition to:

> *consider learning not as a process of socially shared cognition that results in the end in the internalization of knowledge by individuals, but as a process of becoming a member of a sustained community of practice. Developing an identity as a member of a community and becoming knowledgeably skilful are part of the same process, with the former motivating, shaping, and giving meaning to the latter, which it subsumes.* [25]

You are probably a member of several communities of practice. I certainly am. My communities (some of which overlap) include parents, scuba divers, general practitioners, PhD supervisors and people living with and after cancer. For each of these communities, I recall a time when I was not yet a member; a time when I was conscious that I was a novice and keen to learn from others; and a time, often years later, when I was one of the 'old hands' in the community, able to tell the kind of stories that helped other people learn what they needed to know. I have lived my membership of each of those communities both face-to-face and online (in the public domain via Twitter, and privately and sometimes anonymously via closed online communities).

In each of my example communities – whether raising a child, scuba diving, practising medicine, getting graduate students through their PhD studies or living with, and moving beyond, cancer – factual knowledge of the kind you find in written guidance (parenting books, dive manuals, clinical practice guidelines, PhD regulations and patient information leaflets/websites, respectively) gets you only so far. As well as knowing the theory, you also have to know how to *practise* the thing in question. That is why new parents come together to share descriptions of their infants' eating/excreting/sleeping troubles; why scuba divers sit late into the night describing how they survived at depth when the air in their tanks ran low; and why if you get a group of clinicians together, within 5 minutes they will be exchanging stories about 'cases' (i.e. sick patients) and how they handled them. And so on.

As the quote from Jean Lave illustrates, joining a community of practice is partly about acquiring this tacit knowledge – but it is also about *developing an identity* as a member of that community. In clinical communities, the development of professional identity is about the ethical aspects of clinical practice, such as maintaining confidentiality, acting with integrity and what Aristotle called 'case-based reasoning' – that is, making ethical judgements about what is best to do for *this* patient, in *these* circumstances, given a unique set of contingencies. Case-based reasoning needs research evidence, of course, but as every newly-minted junior doctor knows, the evidence (however well you know your randomised trials) does not actually tell you what is the best course of action to offer Mrs Patel, who has glomerulonephritis, in the kidney outpatient clinic on a Thursday morning. That is because managing Mrs Patel is an exercise in professional practice, not an exercise in Bayesian statistics (although the latter may well be brought to bear on the problem).

The difference between the knowledge needed to pass a multiple-choice question on glomerulonephritis and the knowledge needed to offer Mrs Patel professional, ethical care is what you will (hopefully) get from being a member of the community of practice in kidney medicine. Such a community might overlap with a formal, professional society (e.g. people who pay an annual fee and go to conferences on kidney medicine), but the community of practice itself is *informal*. It consists of whoever joins in and is accepted by their peers, and includes both novices who generally keep quiet (or 'lurk', as this is known in online communities) and more seasoned practitioners whose stories contain rich material for learning (and also, occasionally, bullshit – which is why you need a community to contest the knowledge claims rather than just one individual who claims to be a wise old sage and likes the sound of their own voice).

Which brings me to mindlines. 'Mindlines' is a word invented by John Gabbay (a doctor) and André le May (a nurse), academics both, who had

Chapter 10

spent several months observing general practitioners in their surgeries [26]. After carefully analysing their ethnographic and interview data, they concluded that the traditional evidence-into-practice sequence (identify clinical problem → look up research evidence (e.g. in a guideline) → apply evidence) never actually occurred. Rather, clinicians relied on mindlines, which they defined as 'collectively reinforced, internalised, tacit guidelines'. Practitioners developed their mindlines iteratively through browsing journals (often infrequently), informal chats with colleagues, experience from individual patients and discussions with pharmaceutical representatives. In Gabbay and le May's words:

> When describing what we call mindlines, clinicians told us, for example, that they were grown from experience and from people who are trusted; they were 'stored in my head' but could be shared and tested and then internalised through discussion, while leaving room for individual flexibility. Once compiled, each individual practitioner's mindlines were adjusted by checking them out against what was learnt from brief reading or from discussions with colleagues, either within or outside the practice. The mindline might well be modified when applied to an individual patient after discussion and negotiation during the consultation; at this stage patients' ideas of what is the appropriate evidence about their particular case (their own personal history, what their family has experienced, what they have read in the media, and so on) could influence the application or even the continuing development of the mindline. Further adjustment might subsequently happen during swapping stories with colleagues or in audit or 'critical incident meetings'. [26]

These descriptions resonate strongly with other qualitative work on putting knowledge into practice in organisational environments. Van de Ven and Johnson, for example, sum up a wide literature on the practicalities of knowledge utilisation thus: 'users selectively interpret and use knowledge as it serves their own purposes, fits their unique situations, and reflects their relations with their practicing community' [4]. And Huw Davies and colleagues, studying the challenges of applying research knowledge in practice, observe that:

> knowledge use is an elaborate and dynamic process involving complex social processing and unpredictable integration with pre-existing knowledge or expertise. Such integration may require significant unlearning as part of the re-ordering of knowing. [27]

Whilst the difference between abstract knowledge (guidelines) and collectively reinforced tacit guidelines (mindlines) is well described in the social science and philosophy of knowledge literature, it is still poorly understood in EBHC land. Sietse Wieringa and I [28] recently searched the literature for the word 'mindline(s)' and (once we had excluded the work of a researcher whose surname happened to be Mindline) considered what had been written on the topic since Gabbay and le May published their paper.

We found that much subsequent research confirmed that doctors rarely consult written guidelines when making clinical decisions – but that mindlines were in widespread use. In other words, clinicians routinely share and develop their practical knowledge in face-to-face and online communities, citing and challenging written guidelines as they do so. Some authors writing on mindlines acknowledge that there will always be a theory–practice gap when attempting to apply published research evidence to the unique circumstances of an individual patient, but some appear to be living in false hope of a magical day when clinicians will follow guidelines so faithfully and accurately that they will have no need of mindlines [28].

This latter group of authors appear to be aligning with the early evidence-based medicine movement, which explicitly set out to 'de-emphasise intuition, unsystematic clinical experience, and pathophysiologic rationale as sufficient ground for clinical decision-making', whilst stressing the deterministic role of research evidence (especially randomised controlled trials) in clinical decision-making [29]. Although Sackett et al. later softened this stance by talking about the need to integrate best research evidence with clinical expertise [30], Sietse and I concluded that at a philosophical level, much contemporary writing on EBHC continues to rest on a somewhat limited and positivistic view of knowledge as 'facts' that are stored in the heads of individual practitioners and can be immediately and unproblematically applied to clinical cases. If this topic interests you, you might like to look up the counter-arguments we set out in our paper [28].

To sum up this section, clinicians learn much from being members of communities of practice, in which they exchange knowledge with their fellow clinicians. These communities thrive on the knowledge needed for practice – and hence on the practical, case-based and often tacit knowledge that defines clinical experience and expertise. Those who write about EBHC have tended to align with the medical science of epidemiology (trading in the solid, transferable truths of randomised trial evidence) rather than with the social science of healthcare *practice* (in which knowledge is, more often than not, embodied, tacit, dynamic, socially shared and context-bound) Hence, there is still a relatively limited evidence base on how best to support the development of mindlines within professional communities of practice. Along with colleagues in the Netherlands and Norway, Sietse Wieringa and I are working on this challenge, and I hope to update this section with new empirical evidence on mindlines in a later edition of this book.

Chapter 10

10.4 Patient communities and the work of living with illness

In Section 7.3, I introduced the notion of self-management of illness as social practice. By that, I meant that caring for oneself (or for a dependent) with an illness is best thought of not as a set of technical tasks (such as 'weighing', 'calculating', 'using a device', 'consuming medication' and so on) but as a set of activities that happen in the context of a person's lifeworld, and which have both social meaning and moral worth (such as 'keeping in control', 'obeying (or disobeying) the doctor', 'rejecting a gift' and so on). Managing a chronic illness involves a good deal of both practical and emotional work [31], which is typically distributed across a network that includes the patient and his or her family and friends [32].

Mutual support and knowledge exchange amongst people with long-term conditions is not a new phenomenon, but its form is changing. Old-style patient-support groups that met periodically in a local venue, perhaps supported by national or local charities [33,34], have been joined and in many cases superseded by virtual peer-support groups (e.g. on Facebook, Twitter or bespoke online communities that may be independent or supported by a healthcare service provider) [35,36]. The members of such communities value knowledge exchange (both explicit and tacit) as well as practical tips and emotional support [37–40].

The knowledge of how to manage one's own illness overlaps only partially with the knowledge that clinicians draw on to manage diseases; it also includes the embodied, tacit knowledge of particular symptoms and the body's response to treatment [41,42]. Such tacit knowledge is the stuff of communities of practice (which I talked about in the previous section in relation to professional practice), accumulated through years of experience and exchanged through stories [25]. One of my own research interests is the stories that are shared amongst people with diabetes, which convey not merely *what* needs to be done but *how to achieve this in practice* [43–45].

As one of the participants with diabetes interviewed for one of those empirical studies said, 'we learn the facts from you [doctors and nurses], but we learn the meaning from one another' [43]. What he meant by this was that the evidence as presented in conventional patient education – the results of randomised trials of what works in diabetes – was not the kind of knowledge that could be immediately applied in his lifeworld. It had to be re-framed, negotiated and made meaningful through group discussion and story-sharing.

Evidence from patients' tacit knowledge (personally embodied, socially shared) is currently captured poorly if at all in the design of the clinical trials underpinning EBHC, which focus predominantly on discrete 'interventions' that doctors and other health professionals can offer their patients (drugs, operations, specialist technologies, education). Herein lies a paradox: clinician-researchers are building an experimental science of how they can *intervene* in patients' illnesses [46], whilst patients themselves are building collaborative communities aimed at *supporting and informing one another* [37–40]. Hence, I sometimes worry that EBHC's accumulating body of knowledge is growing ever farther from the collective mindlines actually being used by people managing their condition.

Let me give you an example from my own experience. A few years ago, I was diagnosed with breast cancer. Fortunately, it was caught early (stage 1) and treated promptly (with surgery, chemotherapy and a biotech drug called trastuzumab), so my chance of long-term cure was very high (greater than 99%, if you're interested) [47]. But for a few months in 2015, I was a member of a club I had had no desire to join: people receiving chemotherapy. I joined (anonymously, and without admitting that I was a doctor) a social media community on the breast cancer site https://community.breastcancer.org. This is a well-organised site run by moderators that contains numerous topic-based discussion groups. Depending on what you want to talk about, you could join a group on 'newly diagnosed breast cancer', 'dealing with hair loss', 'coping with mastectomy', 'latest research summarised' – or hundreds of other topics.

I was interested in coping with the side effects of chemotherapy. I had already looked up the descriptive epidemiology and found that it was near-universal to experience nausea, and that weight gain (from snacking to relieve nausea) was common and associated with worse all-cause mortality [48]. I had also found randomised trial evidence that taking moderate- to high-intensity exercise every day would reduce my nausea, help prevent weight gain and significantly increase my chance of completing the pre-scribed course of chemotherapy [49].

What I did not know was how to *live* with nausea and loss of taste for 3 months, or how to maintain a strenuous exercise regimen when I felt lousy and had limited motivation. What did I learn from my community of practice that allowed me (as a patient) to implement the evidence I had found in the medical literature? My 'lay' community of practice generated 'mindlines' (see Section 10.3) which reinforced the evidence-based messages, made them meaningful and stressed their importance. People who knew and understood the research evidence fed snippets of it into the discussion (along with web links to research papers). As would be predicted from Section 10.1, there were dissenting voices to the conventional view that chemotherapy (administered as per NICE guidelines) is a good idea, but the overwhelming majority of people in the network bought into this idea and spent a lot of time encouraging their fellow cancer patients to stick their course of treatment.

Chapter 10

We exchanged recipes for menus that seemed to have some taste (if you ever need this information, the food deemed most palatable in my little forum was cheese on toast) and tips for avoiding snacking (a constant temptation when you are nauseous and feeling miserable). And we shared numerous stories of our humble efforts to maintain our exercise levels – often peppered with a dose of humour (since it was hard enough just to make it round the block with the dog, let alone take what we used to call 'exercise'). Again and again we told each other: every little helps. And we also exchanged stories of how our well-meaning doctors kept telling us we must complete the course – but that they had no clue about *how* we were supposed to complete the course.

Another discussion topic in my forum was our doctors' lack of experiential knowledge. Their advice about what something would *feel* like was often seriously incorrect (I shared my oncologist's assurance 'yes of course you'll be fine to go home on the tube after your first dose of chemo' – in reality my husband almost had to carry me to the taxi). These anecdotes affirmed that what we were going through was far tougher than our doctors knew – but also that, week by painful week, we were surviving the ordeal. We counted down the cycles – and we celebrated each member's final infusion, with most posting a picture of themselves hooked up to their last bag of poison. Chemotherapy is so horrible that around one-third of patients default from treatment [50]; in my own breast cancer support forum of around 30 women, nobody admitted doing this except on their doctor's advice after an adverse reaction.

I hope you can see from this example that moral support amongst patients is part and parcel of implementing EBHC, not something separate from it. In describing patient support groups, I have deliberately spoken *as a patient* and used the kind of language that was meaningful to me in my patient role.

I could have written this section differently, focusing on randomised controlled trials in which cancer patients were randomised to 'online peer support on' versus 'online peer support off'. In such studies, peer support via the Internet is depicted as an 'intervention' or 'programme' that doctors provide for their patients (presumably, prescribing it like a drug?). A meta-analysis of such trials, steeped in the language of 'disease management behaviors', 'self-efficacy' and 'medication adherence', pointedly does not mention the problems patients had with their doctors (indeed, none of the included trials had sought to measure any such problems), but expresses its findings thus: 'greater Web 2.0 engagement may be associated with improvements in health behaviors (e.g. physical activity) and health status (e.g. Health-Related Quality of Life)' [51].

Despite the brave attempt to squeeze online patient communities into the 'meta-analysis of randomised controlled trials' box, I am unconvinced that it is valid. Lay networks and online support groups emerge and change organically. They are complex systems that cannot be experimented on or 'controlled for' [52,53]. They exchange the kind of knowledge that is (by definition) hard to define or quantify. As such, they cannot be understood purely through the kinds of research design with which the majority of the EBHC community is familiar. Yet, if it is to remain relevant, EBHC must engage more meaningfully with these communities. In my view, in order to do so, EBHC scholars must learn the language and methodology of the social science of networks and digital communities [54,55], instead of simply doing experiments on them!

10.5 Ten tips for improving networks and networking

1. Extend your definition of what knowledge is
In Section 10.1, I encouraged you to shift your view of knowledge from 'facts' that sit in individuals' heads to framings and understandings (both explicit and tacit) that are developed and shared, and also contested and revised, amongst members of social groups. This collective view of knowledge should help you get your head round what networks are for and why they matter.

2. Revisit the section on how policymakers use evidence
In Section 9.2, I introduced Carol Weiss' taxonomy of how policymakers use evidence. In Section 10.1, I described how disagreement within a network about what is the problem and how it should be addressed will tend to produce a great deal of argumentation amongst the network's members, in which evidence will be continually contested (and multiple versions of it supplied and defended).

3. Know your social influencers
Box 10.2 shows the different kinds of social influencers. These are usually not too difficult to identify. Remember, an opinion leader can lead negatively as well as positively, so if they are spreading misinformation or negative attitudes, they could have serious wrecking power.

4. Note the important principle of homophily
As noted in Section 10.2 (see Box 10.1), a person is more likely to take notice of someone who they feel is like them (e.g. a student nurse might benchmark him/herself against other student nurses; a finance director against other finance directors; and so on). This means that one person's opinion leader is another person's non-entity.

5. Acknowledge social influence as a social process, not an experimental variable

As I explained in Section 10.2, I am not a fan of experimental trials comparing 'opinion leader on' versus 'opinion leader off'. The influence of people in organisations, and particularly of one clinician by another, is a complex social process that is best studied through detailed qualitative work with a naturalistic (real-world) design.

6. Harness the strength of weak ties for spreading ideas

Granovetter's classic paper (described in Section 10.2) is worth reading in the original [12]. The take-home message is that if you are organising networking events, do not just invite the usual suspects who all know each other anyway. Whilst it is harder to organise and orchestrate an event that brings disparate groups from different organisations together (and you will not be able to please everyone, since they will all have different expectations and preferences), you will generally get more bang for your buck if you can pull such an event off. Incidentally, the same principle applies to social media. If you only follow people who hold the same views as you, your social media contacts will be nothing more than an echo-chamber. Be bolder – follow people you disagree with and who do different things in different roles in different organisations and sectors!

7. Support professional communities of practice

Section 10.3 explains the crucial role of communities of practice in the professional learning process. It points out that joining a community is not just about gaining knowledge but also about acquiring an identity. Being an evidence-based practitioner is not merely about what you know but about *who you are*. Professional communities that meet face-to-face still exist, but many operate increasingly in the online environment. They are crucial for supporting the implementation of EBHC (which is why I am researching them).

8. Value mindlines

If you think that mindlines are just a fuzzy, inaccurate version of guidelines, you have not understood what I wrote in Section 10.3. A mindline is to a guideline what 'knowing the ropes' is to a written procedure or manual. Both are necessary – yet the empirical research base on how mindlines emerge and how to influence them is currently sparse. There are plenty more inter-disciplinary PhDs and post-doctoral studies to be done on this topic.

9. Support patient/carer communities

As Section 10.4 emphasised, lay networks, often in online communities, are key to exchanging knowledge and supporting patients and carers living with illness. Such communities have been studied experimentally and their impact measured in terms of biomarkers, health-oriented behaviours (e.g. compliance with medication) and the psychological variable of self-efficacy. I prefer to look at lay support communities as naturally occurring and having their main influence in the lifeworld (i.e. on the complex challenges involved in living with illness in the real world). Whichever perspective you take, there is evidence that they help a lot, and may be key to maximising outcome from evidence-based therapies.

10. Learn from patient/carer communities
In Section 10.4, I gave examples of things I had learnt (as a patient) from joining a community of people with the same illness. If you are a health professional, you might be both humbled and enlightened by the information (often practical, shared through stories) exchanged in online illness support groups on Facebook or bespoke websites. Many will not want you hanging around in their space, but if you put a request politely, you might get invited to see what the expert patients (and newbie lurkers) are up to.

References

1. Hawe, P., Webster, C., & Shiell, A. (2004). A glossary of terms for navigating the field of social network analysis. *Journal of Epidemiology and Community Health*, **58**(12), 971–975.
2. Greenhalgh, T., Robert, G., Macfarlane, F., Bate, P., & Kyriakidou, O. (2004). Diffusion of innovations in service organizations: systematic review and recommendations. *The Milbank Quarterly*, **82**(4), 581–629.
3. Contandriopoulos, D., Lemire, M., Denis, J.L., & Tremblay, É. (2010). Knowledge exchange processes in organizations and policy arenas: a narrative systematic review of the literature. *The Milbank Quarterly*, **88**(4), 444–483.
4. Van de Ven, A.H., & Johnson, P.E. (2006). Knowledge for theory and practice. *Academy of Management Review*, **31**(4), 802–821.
5. Gibbons, M., Limoges, C., Nowotny, H., Schwartzman, S., Scott, P., & Trow, M. (1994). *The New Production of Knowledge: The Dynamics of Science and Research in Contemporary Societies*. London, Sage Publications.
6. Polanyi, M. (1958). *Personal Knowledge: Towards a Post-Critical Philosophy*. Chicago, IL, University of Chicago Press.
7. Star, S.L. (2002). Infrastructure and ethnographic practice: working on the fringes. *Scandinavian Journal of Information Systems*, **14**(2), 6.
8. Friere, P. (1974). *Education for Critical Consciousness*. New York, Continuum.
9. Weiss, C.H. (1979). The many meanings of research utilization. *Public Administration Review*, **39**(5), 426–431.
10. Valente, T.W. (1995). *Network Models of the Diffusion of Innovations*. Cresskill, NJ, Hampton.
11. Rogers, E.M. (2010). *Diffusion of Innovations*, 5th edn. London, Simon and Schuster.

Chapter 10

12. Granovetter, M. (1973). The strength of weak ties. *American Journal of Sociology*, **78**, 1360–1380.
13. Coleman, J.S., Katz, E., & Menzel, H. (1966). *Medical Innovations: A Diffusion Study*. New York, Bobbs-Merrill.
14. Coleman, J.S., Katz, E., & Menzel, H. (1966). *Medical Innovation: A Diffusion Study*. Indianapolis, IN, Bobbs-Merrill.
15. Goldacre, B. (2014). *Bad Pharma: How Drug Companies Mislead Doctors and Harm Patients*. London, Macmillan.
16. O'Brien, M.A., Rogers, S., Jamtvedt, G., Oxman, A.D., Odgaard-Jensen, J., Kristofferson, D.T., et al. (2008). Educational outreach visits: effects on professional practice and health care outcomes. *Cochrane Database of Systematic Reviews*, **4**:CD000409.
17. Flodgren, G., Parmelli, E., Doumit, G., Gattellari, M., O'Brien, M.A., Grimshaw, J., & Eccles, M.P. (2011). Local opinion leaders: effects on professional practice and health care outcomes. *Cochrane Database of Systematic Reviews*, **8**: CD000125.
18. Burt, R.S. (1980). Innovation as a structural interest: rethinking the impact of network position on innovation adoption. *Social Networks*, **2**, 327–355.
19. West, E., Barron, D.N., Dowsett, J., & Newton, J.N. (1999). Hierarchies and cliques in the social networks of health care professionals: implications for the design of dissemination strategies. *Social Science & Medicine*, **48**(5), 633–646.
20. Locock, L., Dopson, S., Chambers, D., & Gabbay, J. (2001). Understanding the role of opinion leaders in improving clinical effectiveness. *Social Science & Medicine*, **53**(6), 745–757.
21. Lupton, D. (2015). The digitised academic. In: D. Lupton (ed.). *Digital Sociology*. New York, Routledge, pp. 66–92.
22. Greenhalgh, T., Robert, G., Bate, P., Kyriakidou, O., & Macfarlane, F. (2005). *Diffusion of Innovations in Health Service Organisations: A Systematic Literature Review*. Oxford, Blackwells.
23. Abrahamson, E. (1991). Managerial fads and fashions: the diffusion and rejection of innovations. *Academy of Management Review*, **16**(3), 586–612.
24. Kaissi, A.A., & Begun, J.W. (2008). Fads, fashions, and bandwagons in health care strategy. *Health Care Management Review*, **33**(2), 94–102.
25. Lave, J. (1991). Situating learning in communities of practice. *Perspectives on Socially Shared Cognition*, **2**, 63–82.
26. Gabbay, J., & May, A.L. (2004). Evidence based guidelines or collectively constructed 'mindlines?' Ethnographic study of knowledge management in primary care. *BMJ*, **329**(7473), 1013.
27. Davies, H., Nutley, S., & Walter, I. (2008). Why 'knowledge transfer' is misconceived for applied social research. *Journal of Health Services Research & Policy*, **13**(3), 188–190.
28. Wieringa, S., & Greenhalgh, T. (2015). 10 years of mindlines: a systematic review and commentary. *Implementation Science*, **10**, 45.
29. Evidence-Based Medicine Working Group (1992). Evidence-based medicine. A new approach to teaching the practice of medicine. *JAMA*, **268**(17), 2420.
30. Sackett, D.L., Rosenberg, W.M., Gray, J.M., Haynes, R.B., & Richardson, W.S. (1996). Evidence based medicine: what it is and what it isn't. *BMJ*, **312**(7023), 71–72.

31. May, C.R., Eton, D.T., Boehmer, K., Gallacher, K., Hunt, K., MacDonald, S., et al. (2014). Rethinking the patient: using Burden of Treatment Theory to understand the changing dynamics of illness. *BMC Health Services Research*, **14**(1), 1.

32. Vassilev, I., Rogers, A., Kennedy, A., & Koetsenruijter, J. (2014). The influence of social networks on self-management support: a metasynthesis. *BMC Public Health*, **14**(1), 1.

33. Ussher, J., Kirsten, L., Butow, P., & Sandoval, M. (2006). What do cancer support groups provide which other supportive relationships do not? The experience of peer support groups for people with cancer. *Social Science & Medicine*, **62**(10), 2565–2576.

34. Kelleher, D. (1994). Self-help groups and their relationship to medicine. In: D. Kelleher, J. Gabe, & G. Williams (eds). *Challenging Medicine*. London, Routledge, pp. 104–121.

35. Eysenbach, G., Powell, J., Englesakis, M., Rizo, C., & Stern, A. (2004). Health related virtual communities and electronic support groups: systematic review of the effects of online peer to peer interactions. *BMJ*, **328**(7449), 1166.

36. Nambisan, P., Gustafson, D.H., Hawkins, R., & Pingree, S. (2014). Social support and responsiveness in online patient communities: impact on service quality perceptions. *Health Expectations*, **19**(1), 87–97.

37. van Uden-Kraan, C.F., Drossaert, C.H., Taal, E., Seydel, E.R., & van de Laar, M.A. (2008). Self-reported differences in empowerment between lurkers and posters in online patient support groups. *Journal of Medical Internet Research*, **10**(2), e18.

38. Wicks, P., Keininger, D.L., Massagli, M.P., de la Loge, C., Brownstein, C., Isojärvi, J., & Heywood, J. (2012). Perceived benefits of sharing health data between people with epilepsy on an online platform. *Epilepsy & Behavior*, **23**(1), 16–23.

39. Wang, Y.-C., Kraut, R., & Levine, J.M. (2012). To stay or leave? The relationship of emotional and informational support to commitment in online health support groups. In: *Proceedings of the ACM 2012 Conference on Computer Supported Cooperative Work*, pp. 833–842.

40. Ziebland, S., Lavie-Ajayi, M., & Lucius-Hoene, G. (2014). The role of the Internet for people with chronic pain: examples from the DIPEx International Project. *British Journal of Pain*, **9**(1), 62–64.

41. Pickard, S., & Rogers, A. (2012). Knowing as practice: self-care in the case of chronic multi-morbidities. *Social Theory & Health*, **10**(2), 101–120.

42. Greenhalgh, T., Wherton, J., Sugarhood, P., Hinder, S., Procter, R., & Stones, R. (2013). What matters to older people with assisted living needs? A phenomenological analysis of the use and non-use of telehealth and telecare. *Social Science & Medicine* (1982), **93**, 86–94.

43. Greenhalgh, T., Collard, A., Campbell-Richards, D., Vijayaraghavan, S., Malik, F., Morris, J., & Claydon, A. (2011). Storylines of self-management: narratives of people with diabetes from a multiethnic inner city population. *Journal of Health Services Research & Policy*, **16**(1), 37–43.

44. Hinder, S., & Greenhalgh, T. (2012). 'This does my head in'. Ethnographic study of self-management by people with diabetes. *BMC Health Services Research*, **12**(1), 83.

Chapter 10

45. Greenhalgh, T., Clinch, M., Afsar, N., Choudhury, Y., Sudra, R., Campbell-Richards, D., et al. (2015). Socio-cultural influences on the behaviour of South Asian women with diabetes in pregnancy: qualitative study using a multi-level theoretical approach. *BMC Medicine*, **13**, 120.

46. Michie, S., Johnston, M., Francis, J., Hardeman, W., & Eccles, M. (2008). From theory to intervention: mapping theoretically derived behavioural determinants to behaviour change techniques. *Applied Psychology*, **57**(4), 660–680.

47. Saadatmand, S., Bretveld, R., Siesling, S., & Tilanus-Linthorst, M.M. (2016). Influence of tumour stage at breast cancer detection on survival in modern times: population based study in 173 797 patients. *BMJ*, **351**, h4901.

48. Playdon, M.C., Bracken, M.B., Sanft, T.B., Ligibel, J.A., Harrigan, M., & Irwin, M.L. (2015). Weight gain after breast cancer diagnosis and all-cause mortality: systematic review and meta-analysis. *Journal of the National Cancer Institute*, **107**(12), djv275.

49. van Waart, H., Stuiver, M.M., van Harten, W.H., Geleijn, E., Kieffer, J.M., Buffart, L.M., et al. (2015). Effect of low-intensity physical activity and moderate-to-high-intensity physical exercise during adjuvant chemotherapy on physical fitness, fatigue, and chemotherapy completion rates: results of the PACES randomized clinical trial. *Journal of Clinical Oncology*, **33**(17), 1918–1927.

50. Chan, C., Wan Ahmad, W., Md Yusof, M., Ho, G., & Krupat, E. (2015). Prevalence and characteristics associated with default of treatment and follow-up in patients with cancer. *European Journal of Cancer Care*, **24**(6), 938–944.

51. Stellefson, M., Chaney, B., Barry, A.E., Chavarria, E., Tennant, B., Walsh-Childers, K., et al. (2013). Web 2.0 chronic disease self-management for older adults: a systematic review. *Journal of Medical Internet Research*, **15**(2), e35.

52. Cohn, S., Clinch, M., Bunn, C., & Stronge, P. (2013). Entangled complexity: why complex interventions are just not complicated enough. *Journal of Health Services Research & Policy*, **18**(1), 40–43.

53. Petticrew, M. (2011). When are complex interventions 'complex'? When are simple interventions 'simple'? *The European Journal of Public Health*, **21**(4), 397–398.

54. Lupton, D. (2015). *Digital Sociology*. New York, Routledge.

55. Wicks, P., Massagli, M., Frost, J., Brownstein, C., Okun, S., Vaughan, T., et al. (2010). Sharing health data for better outcomes on PatientsLikeMe. *Journal of Medical Internet Research*, **12**(2), e19.

Chapter 10

Chapter 11 **Systems**

11.1 Complex (adaptive) systems

Too much of medicine assumes a clockwork universe. We use machine metaphors that reinforce the assumption that we can fix a part of the system as we might fit a new carburettor to a car, and that any new part will slot seamlessly into the old system. One of my sons (an ecologist) once suggested that all doctors – and, he might have added, triallists – would benefit from studying Ecology 101. Such a course would teach them that all parts in a complex system are interconnected – and that you cannot do controlled experiments in a closed system and expect the findings to apply unproblematically to an open system.

Back in 2001, Paul Plsek and I, along with some colleagues, wrote a series of articles for the *British Medical Journal* on complexity theory (not so different from Ecology 101, although my ecologist son might disagree) [1–4]. I will summarise the main points from those articles here.

A complex system (or, to give it its full name, complex adaptive system) is a collection of individual agents who have freedom to act in ways that are not always totally predictable, and whose actions are interconnected. Hence, each agent's actions change the context for other agents. We offered some examples of complex systems in our introductory paper [2]: the immune system, a colony of termites, the financial market and just about any collection of humans (family, committee, primary healthcare team and so on). Such systems have a number of characteristics (Box 11.1).

In subsequent articles in that series, we considered the implications of these principles for the clinical care of patients, for leadership and management, and for education and professional development. In relation to clinical care, and using type 1 diabetes as an example, we argued that because the patient is an agent nested in multiple complex systems, attempting to achieve precise control over the patient's minute-by-minute and day-by-day blood

How to Implement Evidence-Based Healthcare, First Edition. Trisha Greenhalgh.
© 2018 John Wiley & Sons Ltd. Published 2018 by John Wiley & Sons Ltd.

Box 11.1 Characteristics of complex adaptive systems

- **Fuzzy boundaries:** Complex systems typically have fuzzy boundaries – membership can change, and agents can simultaneously be members of several systems.

- **Agents act based on internalised rules that drive action:** These internal rules, expressed as instincts, 'rules of thumb' and mental models, may not be explicit, but it is important to surface them when studying the system.

- **Agents and system are adaptive:** Because the agents within it can change, a complex system can adapt its behaviour over time.

- **Systems are embedded within other systems and co-evolve:** The evolution of one system influences and is influenced by that of other systems. We cannot fully understand the behaviours of agents or systems without reference to the other systems in which they are embedded.

- **Tension and paradox are inherent and cannot be fully resolved:** It is simply not possible to 'fix' bits of a system because creating order in one part may create disorder in another.

- **Inherent non-linearity:** The behaviour of a complex system is often non-linear, which is why it is not possible to predict the weather more than a few days in advance.

- **Unpredictability and emergence:** Interaction amongst parts of a system leads to continually emerging, novel behaviour. Observable actions are more than the sum of their parts. Surprise and creativity are features of a complex system, so the quest for accurate predictability is doomed. Ultimately, the only way to know exactly what a complex system will do is to observe it – it is not a question of better understanding of the agents, better models or more analysis.

- **Inherent patterning:** Despite the lack of detailed predictability, it is often possible to make generally true and practically useful statements about patterns of behaviour in a complex system.

- **Inherent self-organisation:** Each agent acts locally, responding to local feedback on its behaviour – but at a system level, order, innovation and progress can emerge naturally from these interactions. Contrary to what would be predicted in a mechanical system, order may not need to be imposed centrally or from outside.

Chapter 11

glucose level using a carefully worked-out formula (however evidence-based) would ultimately be less successful than aiming for 'good enough' control overall and taking a 'suck it and see' approach to what actually happened to their blood glucose level in the real world [4].

In relation to leadership and management, we made a similar suggestion: instead of tight specification of what should be done when, where and by whom, healthcare would be more efficient and effective if we adopted the principle of minimum specification, allowing local people the autonomy to respond to local contingencies and to decide *how* to deliver on an agreed broad goal [3].

I recalled this article a few years later when I led the evaluation of part of the National Programme for IT (NPfIT) in the UK National Health Service (NHS) [5]. The strategy for NPfIT had been 'ruthless standardisation' and a top-down, centralised implementation programme with rigid milestones, all controlled from an office in Whitehall, where the national director of the programme gazed at a 'dashboard' of aggregated progress metrics. Despite having some of the best brains in the world working on the technologies, the NPfIT went down in some history books as the most expensive IT failure the world has ever known (although the story of its failure was sometimes exaggerated [6]). My team's evaluation (which used both qualitative and quantitative methods) concluded that this reductive, overly specified approach to implementation in a complex system had been a major cause of the programme's demise [7]. As noted in Section 8.4, I recently summarised our main findings for UK policymakers (Box 8.3).

The application of complexity principles to leadership and management partly explains why distributed leadership is a well-established mechanism for dealing with the challenges of organisational change in healthcare [8]. As I pointed out in Section 4.2, distributed leadership does not require one individual to perform all of the essential leadership functions, only a set of people who can perform them collectively [9]. Some leadership functions (e.g. making important decisions) may be shared by several members of a group; some may be allocated to individual members; and a particular function may be performed by different people at different times. The leadership actions of any individual are much less important than the collective leadership provided by members of the organisation.

In relation to learning and professional development, Sarah Fraser and I distinguished between *competence* (what individuals know or are able to do) and *capability* (the extent to which they can adapt to change, generate new knowledge and continue to improve their performance) [1]. We argued that traditional education and training largely focuses on enhancing competence (knowledge, skills and attitudes). In today's complex world, we must educate not merely for competence, but for capability. The latter is enhanced through feedback on performance, the challenge of unfamiliar contexts and the use of non-linear methods such as storytelling and small-group, problem-based learning. Education for capability must focus on process (supporting learners to construct their own learning goals, receive

Chapter 11

feedback, reflect and consolidate) and avoid setting learning objectives with rigid and prescriptive content.

Many years have gone by since I co-authored that early series on complexity. Whilst (in my view) a great deal of talk and writing about evidence-based practice still uses what I call 'Newtonian' language (assuming that a fixed input to a system will produce a fixed output and that the results of interventions can be predicted with some level of precision), there is also a reassuring emergence of papers in which the principles of complex adaptive systems have been applied to implementing evidence.

Top of my list of favourite papers on this topic is Bev Holmes and colleagues' 'Mobilising Knowledge in Complex Health Systems: A Call to Action' [10]. Holmes et al. point out that the principles of complexity theory as just set out are now fairly well known, but few individuals or organisations address these problems optimally. Significantly, 'most health system change initiatives mistakenly attempt to control or manipulate context, rather than foster emergent solutions'.

Drawing partly on a workshop held at the Health Foundation in London in 2015, these authors suggest five principles for the application of complexity theory to knowledge mobilisation (Box 11.2). Perhaps most importantly, they emphasise the value of co-creation approaches, which I covered in Section 6.4, in the context of complex systems.

My list of un-favourite papers in the field of complexity studies includes the work on complex interventions by groups appointed by the UK Medical Research Council (MRC). I should say here that I am unusual in finding this work unexciting (and indeed, in my view, fundamentally misguided); most healthcare academics (including many who sit on panels awarding research grants) consider the MRC's complex interventions framework to be the gold-standard approach for dealing with complexity – so check a few more sources before deciding whether to believe what I am about to tell you.

According to the MRC, a complex intervention comprises multiple elements, all of which seem essential but have 'active ingredients' that may be difficult to specify; they typically operate at multiple levels (individual, team, organisation) [12]. Such interventions include educational interventions, new service models and tests, and treatments that have implications for how services are delivered (e.g. near-patient testing that potentially allows diagnoses to be made in primary care that were previously only possible in secondary care).

Increasingly, health services research consists in developing complex interventions and testing them in randomised controlled trials. The MRC framework proposes five phases (0–4), including developmental and pilot work, the trial itself and an evaluation of post-trial implementation in the real world [13]. Complex intervention trials generally require a cluster design

---

Box 11.2 Principles of knowledge mobilisation in a complex system

- **Leadership is multifaceted and needs to be supported in all its forms:** In a complex system, no one person, group or organisation is able to exercise ultimate authority.
- **Training and development should focus on capability at least as much as competence:** See main text for definitions and rationale.
- **Organisational facilitation of knowledge to action is key:** For planned change to occur in a complex system, actors must play their part – but these actors have a range of accountabilities and responsibilities, allegiances and loyalties, and powers and influences. There may well be perverse incentives and adverse power dynamics. Action at the organisational level (promoting a culture of shared learning, a risk-taking climate and support for creativity) can help overcome these.
- **Change is emergent – and must be treated as such:** In a complex system, it is not possible to predetermine what steps will bring about positive and long-lasting change. Ongoing learning and adaptation across the system are critical to this emergent change.
- **More co-production of knowledge is needed:** Rather than 'Mode 1' (university-led, 'translated' for non-academics), complex systems may see more success with 'Mode 2' research (collaboratively generated by multi-stakeholder systems). See Section 6.4.

Source: Holmes et al. [10] and Greenhalgh & Wieringa [11].

(in which the organisation or service team is the unit of randomisation) and are studied through a pragmatic lens (i.e. seeking to replicate usual care as delivered through the staff and systems in participating organisations) rather than an explanatory one (i.e. seeking to produce abstracted theoretical models of efficacy with an emphasis on scientific purity) [14].

The question that troubles me (and other academics who seek to turn a critical lens on the MRC's work in this area) is whether interventions that are *complex* can be legitimately tested in experimental designs in which they are conceptualised as a clearly defined set of inputs, implemented in a controlled way with attention to mediating and moderating variables [14–16]. I am pretty sure they cannot. Rather, I align with scholars who have argued that the MRC groups may have contributed to the study of *complicatedness* (the study of multiple interacting components in a closed system that behaves according to rational rules) – but that most complex interventions require a more ecological conceptualisation as 'events in systems' and (therefore) a naturalistic rather than an experimental research design to explore their effects [17–19].

Chapter 11

A great example of where such designs might add value is Alex and Matthew Clark's depiction of the Pokémon Go game (which I mentioned in Section 8.3) as a 'supercomplex' intervention in a complex system – and their call for this phenomenon to be investigated using qualitative and mixed-methods research [20].

Complex interventions, as conceptualised by the MRC (i.e. with multiple components but generally delivered to individuals – e.g. a prescription for exercise scheme for people with diabetes), are easier to test in randomised trials than interventions at the level of the community (e.g. increasing access to safe places to exercise) or national economy (e.g. a sugar tax). As I argued in Section 9.2, policymakers are often faced with randomised trial evidence that an individual-level complex intervention is effective (compared to, say, no intervention) but limited evidence (and none from randomised trials) of the effectiveness of population-level interventions.

Emily Oliver and colleagues have recently questioned, from a complex systems perspective, why the evidence base on exercise is so heavily skewed towards individually-focused prescription for exercise programmes whilst we still know almost nothing about the system-level ramifications of introducing widespread promotion of sport and exercise as a public health measure [21]. Their paper beautifully illustrates Alan Shiell and Penny Hawe's plea that instead of developing tighter rules for how to develop a complex *intervention*, we study the complexity of the *system* into which we introduce interventions [22].

One more example. In a paper entitled, 'Why do Evaluations of e-Health Programs Fail?' [23], Jill Russell and I took issue with a paper that proposed the randomised trial as the gold standard for evaluating national IT programmes. Lorraine Catwell and Aziz Sheikh had argued that 'health information systems should be evaluated with the same rigour as a new drug or treatment program, otherwise decisions about future deployments of ICT [information and communication technology] in the health sector may be determined by social, economic, and/or political circumstances, rather than by robust scientific evidence' [24]. Jill and I put forward the opposing view: that e-health interventions (and, most especially, large regional or national IT programmes) cannot be isolated out from the historical, political, socio-cultural and technical conditions in which they emerged and studied as 'pure' scientific interventions with a measurable effect size that is mediated and moderated by a limited number of identifiable contextual variables. We said:

> eHealth 'interventions' may lie in the technical and scientific world, but eHealth dreams, visions, policies, and programs have personal, social, political, and ideological components, and therefore typically prove fuzzy, slippery, and unstable when we seek to define and control them. [23]

Table 11.1 is taken from our paper on why e-health evaluations fail. It contrasts positivist evaluations (based on a mechanistic view of the universe as ultimately predictable and controllable) with what we called 'critical-interpretive evaluations' (based on the principles of complex systems). You can probably see that once you shift from viewing the universe as rational and predictable to viewing it as a complex system, many of the assumptions of what 'quality' scholarship is will need to change.

11.2 Realist evaluation and review

The protagonists of EBHC are sometimes uneasy with the principles of complexity theory introduced in the previous section. It all seems somewhat undisciplined. Whilst they may accept that the world is not as predictable as the philosophy of the randomised controlled trial assumes (after all, why go to all the trouble of nailing an 'effect size' if the finding relates only to the sample studied?), they do not want to abandon the study of what causes what (and with what probability and what impact) altogether. Widely promoted as a way to square the circle is realism, which I will try to explain in this section. I draw heavily on the standards developed in the RAMESES I and II studies led by Geoff Wong and myself [25,26].

The first thing to get clear about realist approaches is that realist evaluations (primary study) and realist reviews (a form of systematic review) are not designed to answer the questions, 'Does this intervention work?', 'What is the effect size?' or 'Is intervention A better than intervention B?' They are done to answer the question, 'What works, for whom, in what circumstances, and why?'

Central to the realist approach is the notion that the same intervention does not have the same impact in different contexts (and indeed, an intervention may have a positive impact in one setting but a negative impact in another – as anyone who has brought up more than one child will know). Hence, the very notion of a transferable 'effect size' or even a confident statement that an intervention 'works' when considering complex interventions in complex systems is nonsense. Also central to the realist approach is the notion of a 'hard' social reality (i.e. social phenomena are real, not just constructions of our minds, and they can be measured – albeit indirectly).

Realist approaches, at least as depicted by Ray Pawson [27], start from the premise that a complex intervention provides some external conditions and resources that can be drawn on by local actors, and that people who introduce complex interventions have (explicitly or implicitly) a *theory of change* as to how those actors will use the resources to achieve an intended change. Realist theories of change focus on what goes on inside people's heads – that is, on what is their conscious or unconscious reasoning (the former may be elucidated by interviews; the latter from observing how they act).

Chapter 11

Table 11.1 Comparison of positivist evaluations (which assume a rational, predictable universe) and critical-interpretivist ones (which assume a complex system).

Positivist studies		Critical-interpretive studies	
Principle	Explanation	Principle	Explanation
1. Overarching principle of statistical inference (relating the sample to the population)	Research is undertaken on a sample that should be adequately powered and statistically representative of the population from which it is drawn	1. Overarching principle of the hermeneutic circle (relating the parts to the whole)	Human understanding is achieved by iterating between the different parts of a phenomenon and the whole that they form
2. Principle of multiple interacting variables	The relationship between input and output variables is affected by numerous mediating and moderating variables, the complete and accurate measurement of which will capture 'context'	2. Principle of contextualisation	Observations are context-bound and only make sense when placed in an interpretive narrative that shows how they emerged from a particular social and historical background
3. Principle of distance	Good research involves a clear separation between researcher and the people and organisations on which research is undertaken	3. Principle of interaction and immersion	Good research involves engagement and dialogue between researcher and research participants, and immersion in the organisational and social context of the study
4. Principle of statistical abstraction and generalisation	Generalisability is achieved by demonstrating precision, accuracy and reproducibility of relationships between variables	4. Principle of theoretical abstraction and generalisation	Generalisability is achieved by relating particular observations and interpretations to a coherent and plausible theoretical model

Principle	Description	Principle	Description
5. Principle of elimination of bias	Good research eliminates bias through robust methodological designs (e.g. randomisation, stratification)	5. Principle of research reflexivity	All research is perspectival. Good research exhibits ongoing reflexivity about how the researchers' own backgrounds, interests and preconceptions affect the questions posed, data gathered and interpretations offered
6. Principle of a single reality amenable to scientific measurement	There is one reality which scientists may access, provided they use the right study designs, methods and instruments	6. Principle of multiple interpretations	All complex social phenomena are open to multiple interpretations. 'Success criteria' and 'findings' will be contested. Good research identifies and explores these multiple 'truths'
7. Principle of empiricism	There is a direct relationship between what is measured and underlying reality, subject to the robustness of the methods and the precision and accuracy of the instruments	7. Principle of critical questioning	The 'truth' is not what it appears to be. Critical questioning may generate insights about hidden political influences and domination. Ethical research includes a duty to ask such questions on behalf of vulnerable or less powerful groups

Source: Greenhalgh & Russell [23]. Copyright: © 2010 Greenhalgh, Russell. Reproduced under Creative Commons Attribution License.

For example, if a country introduces a law to ban smoking in cars containing children, the policymakers implicitly assume that most drivers will reason that it is not worth breaking the law (and hence will not smoke if children are in the car). They may also reason that a change in the law is likely to tip societal attitudes further against smoking in cars with children, thereby putting societal pressure on smokers with children [28]. These theories of change contain mechanisms (processes that operate in some contexts but perhaps not others to generate an outcome) – and it is the link between contexts, mechanisms and outcomes that realist analysis is interested in. In the smoking-in-cars example, such a ban might work better in the United Kingdom (where smoking rates are low and social attitudes against smoking are already negative) than in Russia (where the opposite is still the case and smoking may be strongly linked to cultural identity in some strata of society).

Realist evaluation collects qualitative data (interviews, ethnographic observations and so on) and quantitative data (e.g. waiting times, complication rates, smoking quit rates) and uses them to test hypotheses about which mechanisms operate in which contexts. The use of mixed-method research to develop and test hypotheses about what works for whom in what circumstances is a sophisticated science. If you think you might like to try it, read the RAMESES papers [25,26] and/or Ray Pawson's book [27], or go on an introductory course (at the time of writing, the Universities of Liverpool, Leeds and Oxford all run short courses on this topic; there are also good courses in North America). You could also learn much from the examples of realist evaluations listed in Table 11.2 [8,28-31].

To be honest, I go hot and cold on realist approaches. I have used them myself with some success, but I have also set out with every intention of using them and found myself shifting to a different approach because I struggled to organise my data in the required format of context–mechanism–outcome configurations. I have found the notion of schemas in team learning (see Argyris and Schön in Section 4.3) more useful when looking at change – or lack of change – in organisations. I suspect dyed-in-the-wool realists would say that Argyris and Schön's theories could be expressed in their realist language and tested using realist approaches.

I also part company with Ray Pawson on the question of whether *all* interventions are (in his words) 'theories incarnate', and hence best tested using a 'What works for whom in what circumstances?' question. Perhaps, other framings (e.g. the more open-ended question, 'What happened here and what can we learn from it?', which is what I used to develop an alternative approach to realist review – meta-narrative review [32]) might fit the data better. These arguments have kept social scientists (myself, Ray and many others) deep in conversation until after last orders at conference bars. And they are the subject of another book.

Table 11.2 Examples of realist evaluations and reviews.

Lead author/year	Research question	Context, mechanism(s), outcome	Main findings
Williams 2013 [29] (evaluation)	What works in what circumstances when introducing infection-control intermediaries?	Context: hospital wards Mechanisms: how the intermediary acts; how people react to the intermediary Outcome: improved infection control behaviour	Intermediary presence was associated with change in infection-control behaviour amongst frontline staff. Mechanisms included intermediaries' facilitative approaches to giving feedback and specific teaching strategies. Their success was contingent on prevailing performance management systems, organisational commitment and a learning culture
Rycroft-Malone 2010 [30] (evaluation)	How, why and in what circumstances does protocol-based care work?	Context: different care settings (hospitals, walk-in centres, GP clinics) Mechanisms: how staff interpret and draw upon protocols Outcomes: use of protocols	Protocol-based care works much better in some settings than others. Mechanisms are multiple and context-dependent. For example, in nurse-led walk-in centres, widespread use of protocols allows nurses to practise with a high degree of autonomy; in some medical settings, doctors view protocols as reducing their autonomy
Best 2012 [8] (review)	What works in what circumstances when attempting to achieve large-scale change in health systems?	Context: healthcare system Mechanisms: how policymakers or stakeholders draw on change resources Outcome: system change	Five key mechansims operate differently in different contexts: a. Blend leadership styles (hierarchical with distributed/democratic) b. Establish feedback on performance c. Attend to history/path dependency d. Engage physicians e. Include patients and families in the change process

(Continued)

Table 11.2 (Continued)

Lead author/year	Research question	Context, mechanism(s), outcome	Main findings
Pawson 2011 [31] (review)	What is the evidence for the chain of causation of harm to children when people smoke in cars? To what extent can exposure to harmful toxins be modified?	Context: inside the car Mechanism: biochemical and physiological generation of toxicity Outcome: lung damage	Evidence both for and against smoking bans in cars is contingent (and hence contestable). Chains of causation are complex because the system is complex. Experimental (randomised controlled trial) evidence will be impossible to obtain. Driving with windows open reduces ambient toxins by 90%; partially open reduces toxins by 80%, but levels remain comparable to those in a 'smoky bar'. Whilst not direct proof of harm, this may be enough to inform policy
Wong 2011 [28] (review)	Will a legal ban on smoking in cars carrying children work in a UK context – and why? (Written before such a ban was passed in the United Kingdom)	Context: UK policymaking Mechanisms: how policymakers, members of the public and lobbyists might interpret the (potential) law and what they might do Outcome: law against smoking in cars carrying children is passed and obeyed	When contemplating a change in the law, ask: a. Is the problem likely to be solved by the change in law? (e.g. Will reducing smoking in cars protect children?) b. Will there be public support for the proposed change in law? c. Will powerful lobbyists oppose the law? d. Is it possible to enforce the law in practice?

11.3 Actor-networks

Actor-network theory (ANT) offers a novel view of implementation of EBHC in terms of realignment and stabilisation of a (material and human) actor-network. An actor-network analysis may be particularly appropriate if new technology is a major element in the change effort.

Along with my colleague Rob Stones, and drawing on seminal work by Bruno Latour [33], I have described the key concepts and assumptions of ANT in more detail elsewhere [34]. Briefly, ANT considers networks that are made up of both people and technologies. A key focus is what people and technologies *become* as a result of their position in a network, and the power that emerges from dynamic configurations of human and non-human actors.

Actor-networks are inherently unstable; they require ongoing effort by actors to engage and mobilise their fellow actors (human and technological) in stabilisation work – a process actor-network theorists call *translation* [35]. Stability of the network is always a *truce* of some sort. The extent to which it is ever achieved depends on the degree to which translations are compatible and integrated (convergence of the network) and on the extent to which they can withstand challenge and shape future translations (irreversibility of the network).

Physical artefacts (diagrams, maps, software, infrastructure, objects), protocols and standards help to stabilise a network – but only when these tools and their use in practice are accepted by actors as the way things are and hence no longer questioned ('immutable mobiles') [33]. A clinical guideline, for example, will not stabilise a network unless it is viewed as legitimate and up to date by the various stakeholder groups involved. If that guideline is endorsed by professional bodies and comes to be inscribed in decision-support software, its material presence will aid (although not guarantee) its implementation.

A key concept that originated in ANT but has become more widely used is the notion of the *boundary object* – defined as an object or artefact that is 'both plastic enough to adapt to local needs and [the] constraints of the several parties employing [it], yet robust enough to maintain a common identity across sites' [36]. The boundary object may be key to developing and maintaining stability in multi-stakeholder networks (see Section 11.4), since it can be (to an extent) given different meanings and statuses by different partners in the network but also has sufficient immutability to help align these partners.

Another relevant concept from ANT is unintended consequences. Because actor-networks are heterogeneous and organically evolving open systems, a fixed input will not produce a fixed output. Unintended consequences of innovation feed back to the system in a non-linear way and produce further shifts in the relations between its members (human and technological). Creation of order in one part of the system tends to produce a corresponding disorder in another part [37]. Such phenomena cannot be predicted – they can only be described as they unfold. Some unintended consequences, of course, will be more destabilising of the network than others.

ANT protagonists emphasise that both people and technologies can be thought of as nodes in the network – and that both may be viewed as 'actors'. Technologies 'act', for example, by contributing – as part of a network – to making something happen (e.g. Skype 'acts' by connecting a nurse to her equivalent in another hospital so they can talk). Critics of ANT are quick to point out that technologies do not have agency (i.e. they cannot act) in the same way as humans – but its protagonists depict agency as a *product* of the network, not as something internal to either a person or a technology. In Berg's [38] words:

> *The elements that constitute these networks should not be seen as discrete, well-circumscribed entities with pre-fixed characteristics. Rather, those entities acquire specific characteristics, roles and tasks only as part of a network. A 'physician' is only a 'physician' in the modern western sense because of the network of which s/he is a part and which makes his/ her work and responsibilities a reality…Because of this tight interrelation between elements in a network, the introduction of a new element or the disappearance of an element (as when a hospital stops training junior residents) often reverberates throughout the healthcare practice.* (p. 89)

Studies of the implementation of EBHC from an ANT perspective tend to focus on two main issues: the efforts made by human actors to achieve (or thwart the achievement of) particular alignments of people and technologies; and the tendency of the inbuilt properties of technologies (e.g. access controls or pull-down menus) to shape and constrain the possibilities open to organisational actors. Whilst other research traditions have also addressed these issues, ANT offers a novel way of theorising them. Efforts made by groups of actors to influence the codes, architecture and algorithms inscribed into particular software programmes, for example, are interpreted as *political* moves rather than simple cases of following clinical and technical standards.

Latour has suggested, for example, that if usage of a new technology that aligns with its designers' intentions is a 'programme', resistant individuals seek to mobilise others into enacting and stabilising an 'anti-programme' (in which the technology may be used differently for different purposes), and this wider programme–anti-programme dynamic across the network should be the focus of analysis when studying the non-adoption of a technology.

Here is an example. A recent paper by Alan McDougall and colleagues used ANT to map out the complex and unstable networks of people and technologies that produce action (and, often, a great deal of tension) in the implementation of evidence in the management of heart failure [39]. Heart failure is a physiologically complex and highly unstable state; it involves the presence of too much or too little fluid in different spaces of the body (heart, lungs, peripheral tissues, bloodstream). It also involves the use of multiple technologies to measure where the fluid is (body weight, for example, is a crude but often effective measure of oedema in the tissues; blood pressure is a comparable measure of whether blood volume is adequate; a chest X-ray can detect fluid in the lungs; blood tests for biomarkers can indicate how well the kidneys are functioning) and multiple drugs and procedures to attempt to shift the fluid (e.g. angiotensin-converting enzyme (ACE) inhibitors alter the flow of fluid through the kidneys; diuretics increase excretion of water by the kidneys (ACE inhibitors generally do the same but through different physiological mechanisms); vasodilators take the pressure off the struggling heart muscle).

McDougall et al.'s paper, which is based on extensive qualitative research (interviews and ethnography), puts forward the intriguing suggestion that disputes over the management of heart failure (How much should the patient drink? What dose of diuretic/ACE inhibitor/vasodilator should be given? At what point should dialysis be offered?) are not merely or even primarily a matter of evaluating and applying the body of research evidence (which is complex and contested); rather, such disputes represent a struggle for power and authority amongst different groups of doctors (in this example, cardiologists and nephrologists), who mobilise different combinations of technologies in their efforts to establish a particular account of the evidence as 'facts' in a particular clinical case. Kidney specialists, for example, have control over dialysis machines and the data generated by them (which depict body spaces, and the fluid that occupies them, in relation to the renal system and how it works). Cardiologists, on the other hand, link more closely to echocardiographs, which 'see' the fluid more in terms of what is happening in the heart's chambers. I am oversimplifying (necessarily, since it is a complex paper) – but you might like to look up the original study and explore this actor-network yourself.

The reason I like this paper is that I am currently studying heart failure management myself, but my dataset also includes a community setting where different professional actors (community heart failure nurses, general practitioners) and different technologies (the humble weighing scale and blood pressure machine) are part of the actor-network. Disputes about where the fluid is and how it is best shifted in particular patient cases can be theorised in a similar way – and again, battles about how the problem is to be framed and how humans and technologies are aligned in addressing it are being passionately fought.

Chapter 11

To sum up this section, some concepts from ANT – notably the idea of a dynamic and potentially unstable network involving people and technologies and the notion that a great deal of work is needed to maintain the stability of such an actor-network – are extremely useful in theorising complex change that involves the introduction and use of technologies. My reservation with this approach (which I have set out in detail elsewhere [34]) is that ANT does not include a sophisticated theory of either human agency (embracing, for example, a detailed analysis of what matters to people or how human virtues and vices are brought to bear on actions and interactions) or the macro-social structures in which human action is nested. The quote from Berg earlier in this section suggests that a physician is a physician 'only' because of his or her position in the sociotechnical network – a framing that minimises the importance of such things as professional identity, values and virtues (what some sociologists would call 'agency'). Again, all that is a subject for another book.

11.4 Multi-stakeholder health research systems

This section is about the complex organisational and inter-organisational structures within which research tends to get funded and undertaken these days. Examples include Collaborations for Leadership in Advanced Health Research and Care (CLAHRCs) and Academic Health Sciences Networks (AHSNs) in the United Kingdom – about which, more later.

In Section 9.2, I wrote briefly about the failed Rothschild experiment in the 1970s, where a well-intentioned strategy to align academic research with government policymaking fell flat because of complex practical and cultural differences between the two sectors. In Section 6.4, in relation to citizen involvement with science, and drawing on the work of Gibbons et al. [40], I introduced the notion of 'Mode 2' research, in which the knowledge base is organically co-created *by and with* the intended users of research rather than (as in 'Mode 1') being generated in academic ivory towers and then, in a separate step, 'translated' for its intended users.

Both the failure of Rothschild's natural experiment and emerging evidence from the social science of science (research *on* research) helped drive a complex series of developments in the United Kingdom between the early 1980s and the present day, summarised in Table 11.3 (which I hope nobody will ever require students to memorise for an exam). The story told briefly in Table 11.3 is of a generously funded effort by government, academia and NHS organisations to produce a developed, distributed and accountable research infrastructure that is closely embedded in the clinical work of the NHS and linked to policy through Department of Health funding. Rothschild's simple model of government 'customers' linking to academic 'contractors' was replaced, initially, from 1991, by a systematic R&D (research and development) programme with the aim of generating research relevant to the needs of the NHS [41], and subsequently by a series of ever-more-complex and sophisticated health research *networks* whose stakeholders included service NHS, social care and (latterly) patients and citizens [41–45].

Whilst many scholars consider the direction of travel depicted in Table 11.3 a success [42], the short lifespans of the different bodies and repeated restructurings suggest that the complex system that is contemporary health services research and its implementation in the United Kingdom is neither especially stable nor especially efficient. However, it may well be that it is better than the alternative – which would have been for universities, public-sector health (and social) care and policy to remain in their separate silos. As complexity theory (Section 11.1) suggests, tensions in the system are *inherent*; they need to be managed, not resolved.

Equivalents to the structures listed in Table 11.3 have emerged in many other countries over the past few decades – for example the Canadian Community–University Research Alliances [46], the Dutch Academic Collaborative Centres for Public Health [47] and the Australian Accreditation Collaborative for the Conduct of Research, Evaluation and Designated Investigations through Teamwork (ACCREDIT) [48]. These complex forms should be seen as part of the wider emergence of 'health research systems' – organised networks of researchers, knowledge intermediaries, policymakers and others who provide a context for health sciences research and its uptake and application [41,49]. One recent publication coined the term 'Multi-Stakeholder Health Services Research Collaborations' (M-SHSRCs) to describe their increasingly complex and networked structure [48]. I have chosen to use the term 'systems' instead of 'collaborations' because I am interested in their non-collaboration (what has been termed 'silo behaviour') as well as in their collaboration.

Different scholars have used different approaches to research the operation and evolution of multi-stakeholder health research systems. The detail of such approaches is beyond the scope of this book, but here are some pointers. Harry Scarbrough and colleagues used social network analysis (Section 10.2), along with in-depth qualitative interviews and cognitive mapping, to study the dynamic interactions between UK CLAHRCs [50]. Jo Rycroft-Malone's team used mixed methods (mainly interviews and document analysis) to produce a realist evaluation of a study of CLAHRCs [51]. Ewan Ferlie's team applied critical sociology to consider the complex political interactions needed to make managed research networks (at least partly) governable [52].

The insights generated from such studies are generally highly nuanced and do not lend themselves to simple or universal solutions – but they are nonetheless crucial for improving the support we might offer to such systems.

Chapter 11

Here is an example. In a recent qualitative evaluation of a single CLAHRC, Louise Fitzgerald and Gill Harvey found that governance structures never gelled and that as the programme unfolded, partners began to withdraw their commitment and funding [53]. One reason for this was that once established, the network became divided into silos, each of which became very externally-facing and focused on 'knowledge translation' to audiences beyond the CLAHRC. There was marked duplication of effort and weak internal communication, to the extent that individual teams within the CLAHRC had little idea what other local teams were up to. The authors concluded that externally-facing knowledge translation measures are insufficient to ensure *local* uptake and impact of research findings; attention also needs to be paid to the internal mobilisation and negotiated utilisation of knowledge *within* the network of participating stakeholders – a process they describe as a 'balanced power' form of collaboration.

As Table 11.3 illustrates, one notable policy push in the United Kingdom from 2005 was to align health research with 'wealth creation', especially the outputs of the expanding genomics and biotechnology industries, in what was increasingly referred to as a 'knowledge economy'. In particular, AHSNs, the NHS's 'gateway to the life sciences industry' [54], were developed mainly to support research into, and implementation of, biotechnology innovations.

The 'health and wealth' agenda currently popular in UK research policy rests on Etzkowitz and Leydesdorff's notion of the *triple helix* – that the university sector, industry and government, once separate and independently evolving entities, are increasingly interdependent and co-evolving [55]. In a dynamic and often non-linear process, each sector takes on elements that were traditionally the province of another (e.g. universities develop the capacity to interact with industry and commercialise discoveries; industry develops the capacity to undertake research; and government provides 'public venture capital') whilst also retaining a core identity as academic, commercial and state institutions (respectively).

Central to the triple-helix model is the creation and support of three 'spaces':

1. **The knowledge space:** Collaboration to undertake research and generate new knowledge.
2. **The consensus space:** Building relationships and supporting dialogue amongst university, industry, healthcare staff, policymakers and citizens.
3. **The innovation space:** Collaborations and activities aimed at implementing (and, where appropriate, commercialising) research discoveries, by combining academic or technical expertise with business expertise and (public or private) venture capital.

Table 11.3 Evolution of multi-stakeholder health research systems in the United Kingdom. Drawing on previous summaries [41–45] with additional input from Nick Fahy, Pavel Ovseiko and Glenn Wells.

Date	Milestone
1971	**Rothschild report** proposes 'customer–contractor' relationship between government and science.
1972–78	**'Rothschild experiment'** reveals complex relation between policy and science (see Chapter 9).
1988	**Priorities in Medical Research** (House of Lords Select Committee report) strongly criticises low priority given to research by government (DHSS) and NHS. Calls for investment in research from NHS budget and a National Health Research Authority to fund applied research that will complement MRC funding of basic medical research.
1991	**NHS R&D Programme** established with first Director of R&D for NHS (Michael Peckham). First R&D strategy for NHS, Research for Health, recommends that the NHS spend 1.5% of its budget on R&D, a 'knowledge-based NHS' and development of an NHS-relevant research infrastructure.
1993	**Health Technology Assessment (HTA) Programme** established. Funded directly by Department of Health, with a brief to commission research on the efficacy and cost-effectiveness of tests, treatments and devices that may be used in the NHS.
1994	**Culyer report** (government-commissioned expert task force) proposes that R&D be a core activity of the NHS and that accountability for R&D spend be rigorous and transparent, thereby protecting this key resource stream.
1999	**National Institute for Clinical Excellence (NICE)** established. Its brief is to develop policy in the form of evidence-based guidance on what tests and treatments should be funded, and (later) on how diseases/conditions should be treated.
2004	**UK Clinical Research Collaboration (UKCRC)** established to bring together the NHS, academics, research funders, industry and patients in an environment that facilitates and promotes high-quality clinical research for patient benefit. Seeks to establish **Clinical Research Networks (CRNs)** and **Clinical Trials Units (CTUs)**. Research for Patient Benefit final report (from working party of UKCRC).
2005	**Best Research for Best Health** (Department of Health policy document) makes wide-ranging proposals aimed at meeting the needs of patients and stakeholders. Leads to the creation of the **National Institute for Health Research (NIHR)**. Includes extending and strengthening CRNs, raising the status of clinical researchers and providing new funding streams and centres oriented to applied clinical and health services research.

(Continued)

Table 11.3 (Continued)

Date	Milestone
2006	**National Institute for Health Research** established by Professor Dame Sally Davies. Includes a major capacity-building programme to train applied researchers in primary and secondary care. Key centres include the **NIHR School for Primary Care Research**. Key programmes include the **National Clinical Research Network** (aimed at halting the decline in clinical trials occurring in the United Kingdom) and **NIHR Research for Patient Benefit** (a responsive-mode funding stream that allows frontline clinicians and managers to explore issues emerging in practice). **Cooksey Review** (UK Treasury) reviews publicly funded health research. Endorses reforms proposed in Best Research for Best Health. Emphasises industry's needs and the importance of translational research. Proposes a new **Office of Strategic Coordination of Health Research (OSCHR)**, established in 2007.
2007	**Translational Medicine Board** established to work with MRC and NIHR to coordinate approaches in translational research. First of 12 **Biomedical Research Centres** (BRCs) established to support a critical mass of leading researchers in NHS/university partnerships driving innovation. **High Quality Care for All** ('Darzi review', commissioned by the Department of Health), written by a senior NHS clinician, highlights patchy and slow innovation in the NHS. Introduces a statutory duty of innovation by the NHS. Proposes **Academic Health Science Centres (AHSCs)** – university–NHS partnerships with a focus on discovery and early-phase translation. First **AHSC** established (Imperial College London), initially self-designated and led by Lord Darzi); four more follow in 2009 (all five designated by the Department of Health). **High-Level Report on Clinical Effectiveness** ('Tooke report', commissioned by Department of Health) highlights major gap between evidence and its implementation in the NHS. Recommends a range of measures to promote local ownership of the clinical effectiveness agenda and to increase links between the NHS and university partners – leads to CLAHRCs.
2008	**Collaborations for Leadership in Applied Health Research & Care (CLAHRCs)** established. First cohort of nine CLAHRCs funded by NIHR (with a requirement for matched NHS funding), with the aim of strengthening collaboration between universities and local NHS organisations. The focus is on applied research (much of it community-based) and implementation for patient outcomes.
2009	**NIHR School for Social Care Research** established. Brief to develop the evidence base for adult social care practice. **NIHR Office for Clinical Research Infrastructure (NOCRI)** established to simplify access to the United Kingdom's clinical research infrastructure for the global life sciences industry, with the goal of improving the quality, efficiency and success of translational research.

Year	
2010	**Healthy Lives, Healthy People** (Department of Health policy document) proposes stronger links between public health policy and research, partly via a new **NIHR School for Public Health Research** and a **Policy Research Unit on Behaviour and Health**. The report **Current and Future Role of Technology & Innovation Centres in the UK** makes a case for **Catapult Centres** to close the gap between research findings and development into commercial propositions. In 2011–15, the **Technology Strategy Board** sets up seven Catapults, including the Cell and Gene Therapy Catapult (Guy's Hospital) and Precision Medicine Catapult (Cambridge).
	Establishment of 17 **Health Innovation and Education Clusters (HIECs)**. Partnerships are created between the NHS, higher education, industry and other public and private sector organisations to support the spread and adoption of innovation locally and strengthen professional education and training.
2011	**Innovation, Health and Wealth** (Department of Health policy document) describes research use and innovation in the NHS as 'fragmented, cluttered and confusing'. Recommends closing down several bodies seen as unsuccessful (including NHS Innovation Centre, Institute for Innovation and Improvement, and HIECs) and establishing **Academic Health Sciences Networks (AHSNs)** with a brief to transform health and healthcare by 'putting innovation at the heart of the NHS'.
	A New Pathway for the Regulation and Governance of Health Research (by the Academy of Medical Sciences) notes complex and fragmented structures and variable engagement in research by NHS organisations. Leads to creation of new **Health Research Authority (HRA)** with a brief to promote and protect the interests of patients in health research and streamline the regulation of research.
	Strategy for UK Life Sciences launched by Prime Minister. Sets out a range of measures to support growth in the UK health life science sector. In 2012, Strategy for UK Life Sciences is incorporated into the government's overarching Industrial Strategy with the aim of setting the long-term direction needed to give business the confidence to invest.
2012	**NIHR School for Public Health Research** established. Brief to undertake public health research with an emphasis on what works practically, can be applied across the country and meets the needs of policymakers, practitioners and public.
2013	First **AHSNs** established as membership organisations built on a foundation of healthcare providers and university partners (including some AHSCs), serving populations of 3–5 million. AHSNs extend beyond NHS and academic centres to include community, commercial and third-sector partners.
	Creation of **Local Clinical Research Networks (LCRN)** – a new model for greater local control over funding and resources for supporting research. LCRNs are coterminous with AHSNs, which hopefully promotes tighter coordination between all research and innovation stakeholders in a local/regional context.

Source: [41–44].

A key component of the triple-helix model is the notion of 'new organisational actors' – that is, organisational formats that straddle traditional university–industry–state boundaries – such as incubators, science parks and new models of venture capital (including, for example, social enterprise and patient charities). Indeed, the study of the triple helix may focus fruitfully on the emergence and behaviour of these new organisational actors (e.g. the entrepreneurial university still trains individuals in classrooms, but it also has a more contemporary role of training organisations in incubators).

Importantly, the triple helix rests on an active, questioning civil society, in which public debate over values and scientific priorities and bottom-up initiatives of various kinds feeds into the emergent decisions and actions of macro-level stakeholders (themes that are explored in detail in Chapter 6). The exchange of ideas, knowledge and perspectives is facilitated by free movement of individuals between the different strands of the helix – for example, through placements for students in industry or policy and, conversely, university secondments and honorary lectureships for people from industry, government or the civil service. This in turn depends on reflexivity – that is, ongoing appraisal by the university of its evolving relationships with industry, government and civil society.

Industry, academia, policymakers and the public are traditionally odd bedfellows. Along with my colleagues Pavel Ovseiko and Nick Fahy, and inspired by an idea from my Australian colleague Claire Jackson, I have begun to explore how to apply complexity principles to support Mode 2 research in triple-helix arrangements of Biomedical Research Centres (BRCs). We have adapted Ramaswamy and Ozcan's value co-creation model (see Figure A.11) – a business strategy that engages multiple stakeholders in devising products and services to increase their value for everyone [56]. I explain the adapted value co-creation model in Appendix A.

In sum, the implementation of EBHC has much to gain from the introduction and support of multi-stakeholder health research systems. These are, by definition, large-scale and complex, and they can be researched using a range of different theoretical and empirical approaches. They can be thought of – at least partly – as examples of 'Mode 2' (co-creation) research. And whilst much progress can be attributed to their existence, they are, and will probably remain, imperfect.

11.5 Ten tips for working with complex systems

1. Loosen up

The explanation of what a complex adaptive system is (Section 11.1) should convey to you in no uncertain terms that you cannot predict or control such systems. So don't try. Remember (and I make no apology for repeating this critical sentence from Box 11.1): the only way to know exactly what a complex system will do is to observe it – it is not a question of better understanding of the agents, of better models or of more analysis.

2. Identify simple rules that drive actors
Section 11.1 introduced the concept of simple rules. These are not precise entities but broad drivers of the behaviour of (some of) the agents in a complex system. Get your head round what they are and why they are important – and put work into identifying them.

3. Consider embeddedness
As noted in Section 11.1 and Box 11.1, systems are embedded in other systems. It is tempting (indeed, those of us who have been drilled in the scientific method have a hard-wired instinct) to isolate out parts of the system so as to study them in their pure form without confounders. But in a complex system, the 'confounders' are the whole story. Leave them in – or you will strip away the very things you need to study.

4. When introducing order, look for disorder
Whether you are using a straightforward complex systems lens (Section 11.1), a realist lens (Section 11.2) or an actor-network lens (Section 11.3), you will know that introducing order in one part of a system tends to create disorder in another. If you don't look for these unintended consequences, you will fail to capture them in your analysis.

5. Abandon the quest for a transferable 'effect size'
As Section 11.2 emphasised, the very idea of a transferable measure of how much effect an intervention will have on a system is oxymoronic. Whilst transferable findings from controlled experiments are crucially important (and often valid) in other fields of inquiry, they will give you nothing but false hope if you try to nail them in a complex system.

6. Ask, 'What works for whom in what circumstances?'
Realist inquiry (Section 11.2) may or may not float your boat, but if you are interested in the study of complexity in healthcare you will almost certainly need to get your head round the basics of this approach – if only because the people who give out grant funding are currently very taken with it. Money and study leave to attend a course on the realist approach would be well spent.

7. Map the actors in the network
ANT is another fashionable approach that may or may not appeal to you. Take a look at Section 11.3 and perhaps dig out some empirical studies using

this approach. Have a go at mapping the people, technologies and artefacts in the system you are studying. How are they interlinked – and what moves are key players in making them align in particular ways?

8. Identify boundary objects

As part of your ANT analysis, and to illustrate why this approach can be so powerful, consider the boundary objects (defined in Section 11.3) in the system you are studying. How do different stakeholders interpret and use them differently? How do they serve to bring together people and groups with different priorities and values?

9. Understand the organisational actors in the multi-stakeholder research system

Section 11.4 was probably a hard read, and I never intended Table 11.3 to be committed to memory (or – God forbid – to be used as the basis of examined recall in student assessments). But if you are working in a corner of a multi-stakeholder health research system, it is probably worth your while to understand how the system as a whole emerged, and how the different bits of it fit together. You will play your humble part in it more effectively.

10. Consider how to co-create value for each disparate stakeholder

Section 11.4, on multi-stakeholder systems, is the final section in a book that intentionally became more complex with each passing section. It would be inappropriate to offer a simple fix to such systems as the final piece of advice in this book. If your role is to help support collaborative change efforts in a multi-stakeholder research system, take a look at the value co-creation model in Appendix A (Figure A.11). It is adapted from Ramaswamy and Oczam's value co-creation model for business, and whilst daunting, it may help you to consider how you create different kinds of value and keep your many stakeholders sweet.

References

1. Fraser, S.W., & Greenhalgh, T. (2001). Coping with complexity: educating for capability. *BMJ*, **323**(7316), 799–803.
2. Plsek, P.E., & Greenhalgh, T. (2001). Complexity science: the challenge of complexity in health care. *BMJ*, **323**(7313), 625–628.
3. Plsek, P.E., Wilson, T., & Greenhalgh, T. (2001). Complexity, leadership and management in healthcare organisations. *BMJ*, **323**, 746–749.
4. Wilson, T., Holt, T., & Greenhalgh, T. (2001). Complexity science: complexity and clinical care. *BMJ*, **323**(7314), 685–688.

5. Greenhalgh, T., Stramer, K., Bratan, T., Byrne, E., Russell, J., & Potts, H.W. (2010). Adoption and non-adoption of a shared electronic summary record in England: a mixed-method case study. *BMJ*, **340**, c3111.

6. Greenhalgh, T., & Keen, J. (2013). England's national programme for IT: from contested success claims to exaggerated reports of its death. *BMJ*, **346**, f4130.

7. Greenhalgh, T., Stramer, K., Bratan, T., Byrne, E., Russell, J., Hinder, S., & Potts, H. (2010). *The Devil's in the Detail: Final Report of the Independent Evaluation of the Summary Care Record and HealthSpace Programmes*. London, University College London.

8. Best, A., Greenhalgh, T., Lewis, S., Saul, J.E., Carroll, S., & Bitz, J. (2012). Large-system transformation in health care: a realist review. *The Milbank Quarterly*, **90**(3), 421–456.

9. Bolden, R. (2011). Distributed leadership in organizations: a review of theory and research. *International Journal of Management Reviews*, **13**(3), 251–269.

10. Holmes, B.J., Best, A., Davies, H., Hunter, D., Kelly, M.P., Marshall, M., & Rycroft-Malone, J. (2016). Mobilising knowledge in complex health systems: a call to action. *Evidence & Policy: A Journal of Research, Debate and Practice*. Available from: https://doi.org/10.1332/174426416X14712553750311 (last accessed 14 January 2017).

11. Greenhalgh, T., & Wieringa, S. (2011). Is it time to drop the 'knowledge translation' metaphor? A critical literature review. *Journal of the Royal Society of Medicine*, **104**(12), 501–509.

12. Craig, P., Dieppe, P., Macintyre, S., Michie, S., Nazareth, I., & Petticrew, M. (2008). Developing and evaluating complex interventions: the new Medical Research Council guidance. *BMJ*, **337**, a1655.

13. Campbell, N.C., Murray, E., Darbyshire, J., Emery, J., Farmer, A., Griffiths, F., et al. (2007). Designing and evaluating complex interventions to improve health care. *BMJ*, **334**(7591), 455–459.

14. Eldridge, S., & Kerry, S. (2012). *A Practical Guide to Cluster Randomised Trials in Health Services Research*, vol. 120. Chichester, John Wiley & Sons.

15. Emsley, R., Dunn, G., & White, I.R. (2010). Mediation and moderation of treatment effects in randomised controlled trials of complex interventions. *Statistical Methods in Medical Research*, **19**(3), 237–270.

16. Michie, S., Johnston, M., Francis, J., Hardeman, W., & Eccles, M. (2008). From theory to intervention: mapping theoretically derived behavioural determinants to behaviour change techniques. *Applied Psychology*, **57**(4), 660–680.

17. Blackwood, B., O'Halloran, P., & Porter, S. (2010). On the problems of mixing RCTs with qualitative research: the case of the MRC framework for the evaluation of complex healthcare interventions. *Journal of Research in Nursing*, **15**(6), 511–521.

18. Cohn, S., Clinch, M., Bunn, C., & Stronge, P. (2013). Entangled complexity: why complex interventions are just not complicated enough. *Journal of Health Services Research & Policy*, **18**(1), 40–43.

19. Petticrew, M. (2011). When are complex interventions 'complex'? When are simple interventions 'simple'? *The European Journal of Public Health*, **21**(4), 397–398.

20. Clark, A.M., & Clark, M.T. (2016). *Pokémon Go and Research Qualitative, Mixed Methods Research, and the Supercomplexity of Interventions*. London, Sage Publications.

Chapter 11

21. Oliver, E., Hanson, C., Lindsey, I., & Dodd-Reynolds, C. (2016). Exercise on referral: evidence and complexity at the nexus of public health and sport policy. *International Journal of Sport Policy and Politics*, **8**(4), 731–736.

22. Shiell, A., Hawe, P., & Gold, L. (2008). Complex interventions or complex systems? Implications for health economic evaluation. *BMJ*, **336**(7656), 1281–1283.

23. Greenhalgh, T., & Russell, J. (2010). Why do evaluations of ehealth programs fail? An alternative set of guiding principles. *PLoS Medicine*, **7**(11):e1000360.

24. Catwell, L., & Sheikh, A. (2009). Evaluating eHealth interventions: the need for continuous systemic evaluation. *PLoS Medicine*, **6**(8):e1000126.

25. Wong, G., Greenhalgh, T., Westhorp, G., Buckingham, J., & Pawson, R. (2013). RAMESES publication standards: realist syntheses. *BMC Medicine*, **11**, 21.

26. Wong, G., Westhorp, G., Manzano, A., Greenhalgh, J., Jagosh, J., & Greenhalgh, T. (2016). RAMESES II reporting standards for realist evaluations. *BMC Medicine*, **14**(1), 96.

27. Pawson, R. (2013). *The Science of Evaluation: A Realist Manifesto*. London, Sage Publications.

28. Wong, G., Pawson, R., & Owen, L. (2011). Policy guidance on threats to legislative interventions in public health: a realist synthesis. *BMC Public Health*, **11**, 222.

29. Williams, L., Burton, C., & Rycroft-Malone, J. (2013). What works: a realist evaluation case study of intermediaries in infection control practice. *Journal of Advanced Nursing*, **69**(4), 915–926.

30. Rycroft-Malone, J., Fontenla, M., Bick, D., & Seers, K. (2010). A realistic evaluation: the case of protocol-based care. *Implementation Science*, **5**(1), 1.

31. Pawson, R., Wong, G., & Owen, L. (2011). Myths, facts and conditional truths: what is the evidence on the risks associated with smoking in cars carrying children? *Canadian Medical Association Journal*, **183**(10), E680–E684.

32. Wong, G., Greenhalgh, T., Westhorp, G., Buckingham, J., & Pawson, R. (2013). RAMESES publication standards: meta-narrative reviews. *BMC Medicine*, **11**, 20.

33. Latour, B. (2005). *Reassembling the Social: An Introduction to Actor-Network-Theory*. Oxford, Oxford University Press.

34. Greenhalgh, T., & Stones, R. (2010). Theorising big IT programmes in healthcare: strong structuration theory meets actor-network theory. *Social Science & Medicine*, **70**, 1285–1294.

35. Callon, M. (1986). Some elements of sociology of translation: domestication of the scallops and the fishermen of the St Brieuc Bay. In: J. Law (ed.). *Power, Action and Belief: A New Sociology of Knowledge?* London, Routledge, pp. 196–223.

36. Star, S.L., & Griesemer, J.R. (1989). Institutional ecology, translations' and boundary objects: amateurs and professionals in Berkeley's Museum of Vertebrate Zoology, 1907–39. *Social Studies of Science*, **19**(3), 387–420.

37. Berg, M., & Timmermans, S. (2000). Orders and their others: on the constitution of universalities in medical work. *Configurations*, **8**, 31–61.

38. Berg, M. (1999). Patient care information systems and health care work: a sociotechnical approach. *International Journal of Medical Informatics*, **55**(2), 87–101.

39. McDougall, A., Goldszmidt, M., Kinsella, E., Smith, S., & Lingard, L. (2016). Collaboration and entanglement: an actor-network theory analysis of team-based

intraprofessional care for patients with advanced heart failure. *Social Science & Medicine*, **164**, 108–117.

40. Gibbons, M., Limoges, C., Nowotny, H., Schwartzman, S., Scott, P., & Trow, M. (1994). *The New Production of Knowledge: The Dynamics of Science and Research in Contemporary Societies*. London, Sage Publications.

41. Hanney, S., Kuruvilla, S., Soper, B., & Mays, N. (2010). Who needs what from a national health research system: lessons from reforms to the English Department of Health's R&D system. *Health Research Policy and Systems*, **8**, 11.

42. Walshe, K., & Davies, H.T. (2013). Health research, development and innovation in England from 1988 to 2013: from research production to knowledge mobilization. *Journal of Health Services Research & Policy*, **18**(3 Suppl.), 1–12.

43. Shaw, S.E., & Greenhalgh, T. (2008). Best research – for what? Best health – for whom? A critical exploration of primary care research using discourse analysis. *Social Science & Medicine*, **66**(12), 2506–2519.

44. Ovseiko, P.V., O'Sullivan, C., Powell, S.C., Davies, S.M., & Buchan, A.M. (2014). Implementation of collaborative governance in cross-sector innovation and education networks: evidence from the National Health Service in England. *BMC Health Services Research*, **14**(1), 1.

45. Shergold, M., & Grant, J. (2008). Freedom and need: the evolution of public strategy for biomedical and health research in England. *Health Research Policy and Systems*, **6**(1), 1.

46. King, G., Servais, M., Forchuk, C., Chalmers, H., Currie, M., Law, M., et al. (2010). Features and impacts of five multidisciplinary community-university research partnerships. *Health and Social Care in the Community*, **18**(1), 59–69.

47. Wehrens, R., Bekker, M., & Bal, R. (2014). Hybrid management configurations in joint research. *Science, Technology & Human Values*, **39**(1), 6–41.

48. Hinchcliff, R., Greenfield, D., & Braithwaite, J. (2014). Is it worth engaging in multi-stakeholder health services research collaborations? Reflections on key benefits, challenges and enabling mechanisms. *International Journal for Quality in Health Care*, **26**(2), 124–128.

49. Hanney, S., Gonzalez-Block, M.A., Buxton, M.J., & Kogan, M. (2003). The utilisation of health research in policy-making: concepts, examples and methods of assessment. *Health Research Policy and Systems*, **1**(1), 2.

50. Scarbrough, H., D'Andreta, D., Evans, S., Marabelli, M., Newell, S., Powell, J., & Swan, J. (2014). Networked innovation in the health sector: comparative qualitative study of the role of Collaborations for Leadership in Applied Health Research and Care in translating research into practice. *Health Services and Delivery Research*, **2**, 13.

51. Rycroft-Malone, J., Burton, C., Wilkinson, J., Harvey, G., McCormack, B., Baker, R., et al. (2015). Collective action for knowledge mobilisation: a realist evaluation of the Collaborations for Leadership in Applied Health Research and Care. *Health Services and Delivery Research*, **3**, 44.

52. Ferlie, E. (2013). *Making Wicked Problems Governable? The Case of Managed Networks in Health Care*. Oxford, Oxford University Press.

53. Fitzgerald, L., & Harvey, G. (2015). Translational networks in healthcare? Evidence on the design and initiation of organizational networks for knowledge mobilization. *Social Science & Medicine*, **138**, 192–200.

54. McGough, R., & Rubenstein, S. (2013). Academia. Shaping the new science networks. *Health Service Journal*, **123**(6340), 32–33.
55. Etzkowitz, H., & Leydesdorff, L. (2000). The dynamics of innovation: from National Systems and 'Mode 2' to a Triple Helix of university–industry–government relations. *Research Policy*, **29**(2), 109–123.
56. Ramaswamy, V., & Ozcan, K. (2014). The co-creation paradigm. Stanford, CT, Stanford University Press.

Appendix A **Frameworks, tools and techniques**

Recall what I said in Section 1.2: there is no tooth fairy. The evidence-based healthcare (EBHC) movement has set much store by methods, tools and protocols, but implementing evidence is not something that can be tightly pre-specified and 'blueprinted'. It follows that the quest to produce a conceptual or analytic framework to guide the implementation of evidence will never produce anything more than one person's (or one group's) perspective on that challenge. As Cathy Howe recently quoted (citing an apocryphal story whose original author is untraceable), 'Frameworks are like toothbrushes: everyone's got one, and no-one wants to use anyone else's'.

In this appendix, I offer an eclectic (and inevitably incomplete) selection of frameworks, tools and techniques that may help with the practical task of implementation. Please suggest additional frameworks that you think would fit into this appendix – they may appear in a subsequent edition!

Some of the frameworks here were developed specifically to support the introduction of new, evidence-based ideas and practices. Others have been borrowed from the quality-improvement literature. Many of the tools are ubiquitous in the literature and have been published and republished in different forms over the years, making it impossible to trace the original copyright of the idea or model. Where I could, I have acknowledged an original source. None of them are my own ideas, although I have adapted some for clarity.

I draw on compilations by others, including the Institute for Health Improvement (IHI) in the United States, the Canadian Institute for Health Sciences (CAHS), the King's Fund and NHS Scotland in the United Kingdom, as well as Cathy Howe et al.'s review article on the tools and techniques that were used to support improvement work in a quality collaborative [1]. I am also grateful to Louise Locock for permission to plunder an (unpublished) handbook of quality-improvement models and tools that she compiled for the National Institute for Health Research (NIHR)-funded UsPEX research

How to Implement Evidence-Based Healthcare, First Edition. Trisha Greenhalgh.
© 2018 John Wiley & Sons Ltd. Published 2018 by John Wiley & Sons Ltd.

study (in which I play a small part). Whilst the models in that handbook are not Louise's own, the work she did to collate and summarise them was considerable.

Care bundles

A care bundle is *a small set of evidence-based interventions for a defined patient population and care setting* [2]. The concept came originally from the IHI in 2001; an update in 2012 explains their history and rationale [2]. The initial goal was to reduce variation in care outcomes in high-risk clinical situations such as ventilated patients on intensive care units, but the concept of a bundle has spread much more widely. The initial 'IHI Ventilator Bundle' consisted of the following evidence-based steps:

- elevation of the head of the bed to between 30 and 45°;
- daily 'sedation vacations' and assessment of readiness to extubate;
- peptic ulcer disease (PUD) prophylaxis;
- deep venous thrombosis (DVT) prophylaxis;
- (a fifth bundle element, 'daily oral care with chlorhexidine,' was added in 2010).

The care bundle adds value because (and to the extent that) it aligns a collection of tasks that can be implemented and audited together, allowing a multidisciplinary team to pull together and consider how they will deliver the bundle as a whole. As the IHI report [2] states:

> when compliance is measured for a core set of accepted elements of care for a clinical process, the necessary teamwork and cooperation required will result in high levels of sustained performance [reliability] not observed when working to improve individual elements. (p. 4)

The IHI guidelines for preparing care bundles are shown in Box A.1. Importantly, care bundles are about tasks and interventions that are *already agreed upon* by participating teams and team members. If your problem is that local clinicians dispute the evidence, you need to start somewhere else (perhaps PARIHS).

Care bundles do not implement themselves. Other tools and approaches listed in this appendix may help in this regard (e.g. process mapping, PDSA, measuring for improvement). Remember, as in all improvement efforts, patients and carers may be important partners in the design, implementation and evaluation of a care bundle. There is no set formula – so be creative and tap into local knowledge.

> **Box A.1 Institute for Health Improvement (IHI) guidelines**
> **for designing care bundles**
> - The bundle has three to five interventions (elements), with strong clinician agreement.
> - Each bundle element is relatively independent.
> - The bundle is used with a defined patient population in one location.
> - The multidisciplinary care team develops the bundle.
> - Bundle elements should be descriptive rather than prescriptive, to allow for local customisation and appropriate clinical judgement.
> - Compliance with bundles is measured using all-or-none measurement, with a goal of 95% or greater.
>
> *Source: Reproduced from [2].*

Laura Lennox's team in London explored the challenges of implementing care bundles for chronic obstructive pulmonary disease (COPD) [3]. They classified these challenges under five dimensions: staffing, infrastructure, process, use of improvement methodology and patient and public involvement. These headers might serve as a good framework of things to think about when setting out to design a care bundle.

Driver diagrams

A driver diagram (to use the King's Fund definition) is *a conceptual model that helps teams to identify an aim they want to achieve and then to align the relevant system components in order to support its achievement.* There are two aspects to a driver diagram: product and process. Personally, I am more interested in the latter.

The driver diagram is a diagram depicting team members' current shared theories of 'cause and effect' in the system. It is usually produced with a lot of arguing, negotiating, white-boarding, flip-charting and putting sticky notes on walls. This is the (messy, interactive, dynamic) *process* of driver diagramming. The diagram (product) is rarely if ever a perfect summary of what everyone thinks – but the diagramming (process) serves the important function of organisational sense-making (see Section 5.5).

Driver diagramming sets the stage for defining the 'how' elements of a project – the specific changes or interventions that will lead to the desired outcome. It helps to define which aspects of the system should be measured and monitored – both in terms of outcomes (to see if the interventions are effective) and in terms of theories of change (to test whether the causal theories proposed at the outset actually explain the project's successes, failures and things in between). Driver diagramming also helps a team clarify and

Appendix A

(hopefully) reach agreement on the aim and scope of the work and provides a forum for generating ideas for refining and delivering the intervention. Driver diagramming and process mapping (see later) are closely linked and should be used together.

A template for a driver diagram is shown in Figure A.1. The King's Fund provides an excellent resource with more information on driver diagrams and driver diagramming [4].

Experience-Based Co-Design (EBCD)

Originally developed by Paul Bate and Glenn Robert [6] and operationalised by the King's Fund, which has produced an extensive online manual and resource kit [7], EBCD seeks *to ensure that health services and/or care pathways are designed and continually redesigned around the subjective experiences of patients and carers.*

The King's Fund online manual describes the process thus:

> *[EBCD] involves gathering experiences from patients and staff through in-depth interviewing, observations and group discussions, identifying key 'touch points' (emotionally significant points) and assigning positive or negative feelings. A short edited film is created from the patient interviews. This is shown to staff and patients, conveying in an impactful way about how patients experience the service. Staff and patients are then brought together to explore the findings and to work in small groups to identify and implement activities that will improve the service or the care pathway.* [7]

The detail of how to do this in practice (e.g. how to recruit a representative sample of patients; how to run the patient groups; how to make a film to convey the key touch points) is described on the King's Fund website (www.kingsfund.org.uk). There is even a section entitled 'Adapting the EBCD Approach to Your Budget'.

As an academic, I am interested in the underlying conceptual and theoretical basis of EBCD, which includes:

- a grounding in phenomenology (the starting point for analysis and improvement effort is data on the *subjective* perceptions, experiences and emotional reactions of the individual patient, carer and frontline staff member, not 'objective' data such as waiting times);
- a strong focus on *pragmatic application* of the approach to frontline health and care services;
- the use of *collective sense-making* (see Section 5.5) and negotiation to produce 'new understandings, relationships, and engagements' [8].

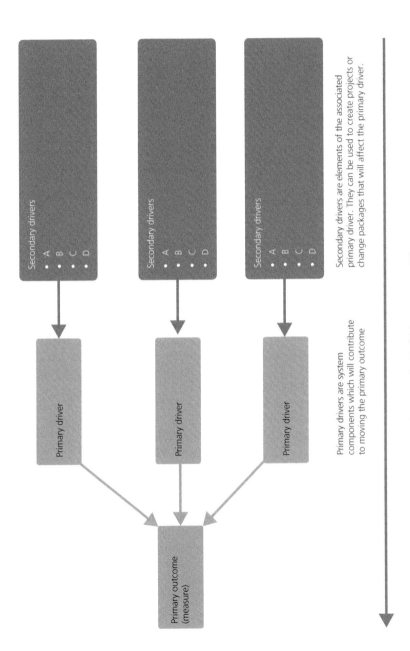

Figure A.1 Template for a driver diagram. *Source:* US Institute for Health Improvement [5].

The question of how EBCD aligns with implementation of EBHC is not straightforward. Theoretically, patients (or indeed staff) might redesign the service in a way that gave everyone a warm feeling inside but ultimately led to (say) more deaths or less efficient use of resources. There are two arguments against such an eventuality. First, EBCD has been around a long time and there are no examples yet of such an eventuality occurring. Second, the co-design process is a process of dialogue – and reservations about the direction of the discussion can be fed into the collective deliberations of the redesign process. There is a research study waiting to be done that explicitly seeks to align the experience-based evidence of EBCD with the objective evidence from published research and test the null hypothesis that these streams of evidence cannot be aligned.

Knowledge-to-Action (KTA) framework

The KTA framework was first set out in a paper by Ian Graham and colleagues entitled 'Lost in Knowledge Translation: Time for a Map?' [9]. It is reproduced in Figure A.2.

The centrepiece of the KTA model is what Graham and colleagues call the 'knowledge funnel' – a process by which knowledge is surfaced, synthesised and tailored to particular audiences (see Section 2.5 for my own suggestions on how to achieve the tailoring and shaping work of knowledge translation). Around the outside is a continuous, iterative 'action cycle' of: identifying problems; selecting suitable tailored knowledge for each problem; adapting the selected knowledge to the local context; identifying local barriers to the uptake and use of this knowledge; selecting and tailoring interventions to overcome these barriers (and thus promote and support knowledge use); monitoring knowledge use; evaluating outcomes; and sustaining knowledge use.

My students find the KTA framework very useful for getting started in real-world EBHC implementation projects. It is certainly a very good way to start if the task is to write an essay about a particular knowledge-translation challenge in a particular group, team or small organisation. It reminds us that the knowledge from research studies needs to go through a 'funnel' before it is likely to be meaningful or useful to frontline service staff. It also reminds us that both the outcomes of the EBHC implementation effort and the continuation/sustainability of knowledge use need to be systematically monitored.

My reservation about this framework is that it is an example of a 'barriers and facilitators' approach (see Sections 9.1, 9.2 and 10.1). To recap, whilst

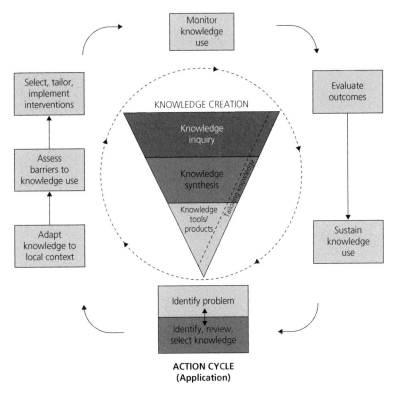

Figure A.2   The Knowledge-to-Action (KTA) framework. *Source:* Graham et al. [9].

identifying barriers and potential facilitators to the uptake of knowledge can be useful up to a point, such frameworks tend to be based on an 'evidence-centric' and overly rational view of knowledge use. They can overlook the complex ways in which knowledge (including but not limited to research knowledge) is actually generated, exchanged and used in practice.

My advice is: use the KTA framework to get you started. If it works well, fine. But if you find yourself struggling to fit your messy real-world situation into the diagram in Figure A.2, it may be worth revisiting the sections where I present less 'rational' perspectives on what knowledge is and how it is used. See for example Carol Weiss's taxonomy of the many ways in which knowledge is utilised in policymaking (Section 9.2), Damien Contandriopoulos and colleagues' systematic review of knowledge use (Section 10.1) and Gabbay and le May's description of professional mindlines (Section 10.3).

Measuring for improvement

One of my favourite resources on measuring for quality improvement is the website of the Quality Improvement Hub of NHS Scotland [10]. There are many other similar websites offering identical or similar versions of the same tools and resources. To quote from NHS Scotland:

> *The aim of improvement endeavours in healthcare is to make services better. That might be safer (less errors, infections, falls), more effective (delivering care that is based on science – neither over or under treating), more efficient (less waste), more person-centred (caring, compassionate, fitting with patient/family requests), equitable or timely.*
>
> *To understand whether we have reached our aims we need to define what our chosen 'better' state would look like and measure things to know if the changes we make result in the improvements we seek.*
>
> *Measurement for improvement asks questions like:*
>
> - *What does 'better' look like?*
> - *How will we recognise better when we see it?*
> - *How do we know if a change is an improvement?*
>
> *Data and measurement is required:*
>
> - *To plan for improvement*
> - *For testing changes*
> - *For tracking compliance*
> - *For determining outcomes*
> - *For monitoring long term progress*
> - *To make improvement visible and tell an improvement story.* [10]

The site also quotes Kaplan and Norton's seminal paper, 'The Balanced Scorecard': 'The use of measurement as a language helps translate complex and frequently nebulous concepts into a more precise form …' [11]. The downside of focusing on measurement and measuring what can (easily) be measured diverts our attention from other, equally important things that are difficult or impossible to measure. But this does *not* mean that we should give up on measuring anything – it just means that we should use measurement to inform our judgements, not as a substitute for those judgements.

The steps involved in measurement for improvement are shown schematically in Figure A.3. You can see that a highly rational process of setting aims, defining concepts, establishing and refining measures and so on is depicted. If you have ever tried this, you will know it is rarely this neat (or politically

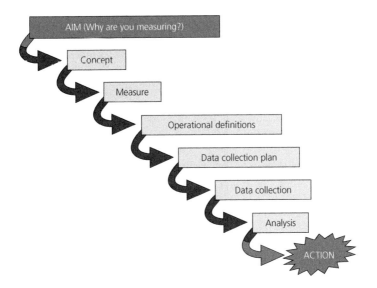

Figure A.3   Schematic diagram of measurement for improvement. *Source:* NHS Scotland [10]. Taken from Lloyd, R. (2004). *Quality Health Care: A Guide to Developing and Using Indicators.* Burlington, MA, Jones & Bartlett.

uncontentious) in practice! The metrics and measures actually used will be a compromise between what you would like to measure (from a theoretical perspective), what key stakeholders will allow you to measure and what you have the resources (time, money, instruments) to measure.

Almost everyone sets out to measure too many things, too frequently, paying too little attention to whether the data will be usable and with insufficient man/womanpower to analyse the data and feed them back into the improvement cycle. My tip: measure fewer things, less frequently; select the kinds of measure that frontline staff will find meaningful and useful in driving improvement; use routinely collected data as much as possible; and assign your resources to ensuring that the feedback cycle is closed as tightly as possible (see Chapter 11 for why this is important).

The term 'data' in Figure A.3 can of course mean either quantitative or qualitative data – or, indeed, a combination of the two. Quantitative measures can be simple descriptive statistics that you can generate readily without specialist help (e.g. 'did not attend' rates or the percentage of respondents agreeing with a yes/no question in a survey). They can also include more advanced tools such as demand and capacity analysis or statistical process control charts. These are not as terrifying or as impossible as they may sound – see NHS Scotland's guide for some techniques and examples [10].

Qualitative data for measurement of improvement can include free-text responses in surveys, interviews (semi-structured or narrative), focus groups and the products of group activities such as writing sticky notes and grouping them on a wall. The NHS Scotland and King's Fund websites (and many others) give further details of what these approaches are and how to apply them in practice.

Both quantitative and qualitative measurement data can be generated from a valid (trustworthy) sample or from a biased (skewed, unrepresentative) one. Many patients who are asked by a powerful person (e.g. their doctor) to fill out a survey or tell a story about their experience are unlikely to raise everything that might be troubling them (see Section 7.4 for an explanation of why not). If you do not take account of these important issues when designing and using your quality improvement measures, you will be able to do little more than demonstrate the validity of the old maxim 'garbage in, garbage out'.

NHS Institute for Innovation and Improvement (NHS III) Sustainability Model

It is a sad irony that the NHS institute that supported the follow-through of quality-improvement efforts in the long term, with a focus on their sustainability, was closed down in 2013. I was a great fan of the NHS III. Its 'Sustainability Guide' defines sustainability as *when new ways of working and improved outcomes become the norm*: 'Not only have the process and outcome changed, but the thinking and attitudes behind them are fundamentally altered and the systems surrounding them are transformed as well' [12].

Achieving sustained improvement is much tougher than demonstrating a short-term gain that may slide back when people's attention moves on to a new project or different deadline. The Sustainability Model (Figure A.4) is a diagrammatic aide-memoire to help teams consider the people, processes and organisational elements needed to support the introduction, routinisation and sustainability of an improvement effort – and give particular attention to factors that might affect the initiative's long-term success.

Process elements in the NHS III Sustainability Model include communicating the evidence for a change to staff in a way they find credible; encouraging staff to consider the benefits of the proposed change beyond helping patients (e.g. would it make their jobs easier?); adapting the intervention over time to take account of local contingencies; and ensuring the effectiveness of the system to monitor progress (see 'Measuring for Improvement').

The 'staff' dimension of this model reminds us to consider the crucial role of senior leaders (top management and what I would call 'expert opinion leaders' – see Section 4.2 on leadership and Section 10.2 on social

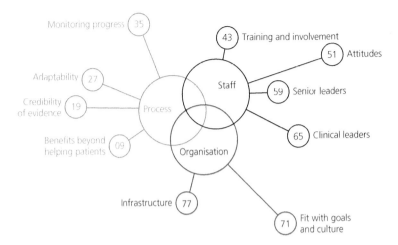

Figure A.4 NHS III Sustainability Model. *Source:* NHS Institute for Innovation and Improvement [12]. Reproduced with permission of NHS England.

influencers) and clinical leaders (I would call these 'peer opinion leaders' and 'champions' – Section 10.2), and also to attend to staff training and staff attitudes (the theoretical dimensions of these influences are covered in Sections 3.2, 4.3, 5.5 and 5.6).

The 'organisational' elements of this model are twofold: infrastructure (both 'hard', such as job descriptions, policies and procedures, and 'soft', such as communication and attention to staff concerns) and fit with organisational goals and culture (if there isn't much, your job will be much harder). These elements map on to several components of the diffusion of innovations model described in Chapter 5.

In sum, the NHS III Sustainability Model is beginning to pop up in the academic and (more so) the 'grey' literature on implementing EBHC. Whilst the components highlighted have all been shown to be significant influences on the success and sustainability of change efforts, as described elsewhere in this book, I am somewhat alarmed that this model is sometimes referred to as 'the ten factors of sustainability' (as if all you need to do is tick off each 'factor' without understanding the theoretical basis of why that particular factor is key to the model or how it fits with all the other factors).

My advice: if Figure A.4 helps you apply the theoretical concepts you have read about elsewhere in this book to a real EBHC implementation scenario, do use it. But I personally think it is more of an aide-memoire for the implementation process than a tool for achieving sustainability (for a more theoretical take on the latter, see Section 5.6).

Public Involvement Impact Assessment Framework (PIIAF)

Developed by a team based at the Universities of Lancaster, Liverpool and Exeter and led by Jennie Popay, PIIAF offers a theory-informed way of assessing the impact of citizen involvement in the research process. I discuss it briefly in Section 6.2, where I talk about the importance of making values explicit.

PIIAF has two components, which I have called *groundwork* (considering all the issues that can shape the impact of public involvement: Figure A.5) and *developing an impact assessment plan* (Figure A.6). The framework is intended to be used flexibly and creatively, rather than as a rigid set of steps.

In relation to groundwork, the four elements around the circle (values, approaches, research focus and study design, and practicalities) in Figure A.5 will all be mutually dependent and co-evolving. There may be historical or organisational reasons why things need to be done (or cannot be done) in a

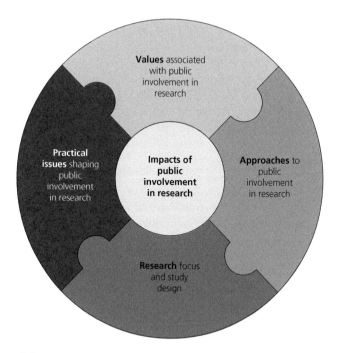

Figure A.5 Issues to consider when involving the public in research. *Source:* Part of the Public Involvement Impact Assessment Framework (PIIAF). Popay & Collins [13]. Reproduced with permission of Popay & Collins.

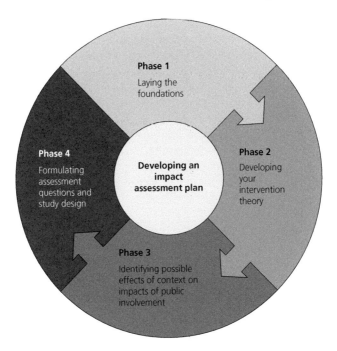

Figure A.6 Developing an impact assessment plan for public involvement in research. *Source:* Part of the Public Involvement Impact Assessment Framework (PIIAF). Popay & Collins [13]. Reproduced with permission of Popay & Collins.

particular way. Particular resources may have to be spent on particular things – and so on. Hence, there is no formula for how these broad issues should be mapped out and considered. Rather, PIIAF provides a set of questions under each heading to inform discussions within research teams. These questions and the headings can be used in setting the agendas for meetings (and deciding who to invite), collecting preliminary data (perhaps through interviews or brainstorming with flip-charts or sticky notes), researching what has happened to date (perhaps by collecting documents such as annual reports or current job descriptions) and guiding conversations amongst stakeholders.

The PIIAF guide (freely available as a download) and the PIIAF website (www.piiaf.org.uk) offer more detail, as well as some resources for running interactive meetings (such as cards to prompt discussion). One important message is that the results of all this groundwork should be recorded in a clear summary, preferably structured according to the four 'issues' headers in Figure A.5. You can download a blank record card from the PIIAF website to help with this.

In relation to developing the plan for assessing impact, Figure A.6 shows a cycle that must be grown organically, giving attention to multiple competing issues and values (see Section 6.2). Evaluation of public involvement would generally need to include formative elements (feedback loops to tell people how things are going – see 'PDSA Cycles'), process elements (assessment of environmental drivers, barriers and tricky issues – sometimes written up as a case narrative with illustrative examples) and summative elements (specific measures and metrics of success, usually defined in advance as part of a logic model). The section on 'Measurement for Improvement' is also relevant to the evaluation of citizen involvement.

Taking the steps in Figure A.6 in turn, you need to consider the following:

1. Laying the foundations:
   * *Why* do you want to assess the impact of public involvement in your research?
   * *Who* should be involved (and how) in the design and conduct of the impact assessment?
2. Developing your intervention theory:
   * *How* (i.e. through what causal pathways) will your approach to citizen involvement lead to the impacts you are seeking? Consider, for example, that there may be multiple pathways between involving citizens and achieving outcomes; that different stakeholders may have different ideas about these pathways; that involvement may have unintended consequences – positive and negative; and that attribution (i.e. saying for sure that X *caused* Y) may be difficult or impossible because of the multiple interacting variables in a complex system.
3. Influence of context:
   * How might the *context* in which your research will take place affect the process of public involvement and/or its impacts? Context can include the research focus and study design; values and behaviours in the research team and in wider setting or organisation; and practical issues including structures, procedures and resources.
4. Formulating assessment questions and developing the assessment. This final phase of planning consolidates the data from the previous three steps and sharpens the focus:
   * *What specific questions* do you want your impact assessment to answer?
   * *What approach* to impact assessment will you use?
   * *What specific data* will you need to collect and how will you do this?
   * *What challenges* will you need to address and which might limit what is feasible?

As with all evaluations, assessing the impact of citizen involvement needs to be realistic and achievable within the resources and timeframe of your project.

I strongly recommend that you explore the PIIAF website for tools to guide you through this important aspect of implementing EBHC.

Promoting Action on Research Implementation in Health Services (PARIHS)

PARIHS is a conceptual model describing the implementation of research in practice. It depicts the successful implementation of research as dependent on the interplay between three core elements:

1. the strength, nature and plausiblity of the *evidence* to be used;
2. the *context or environment* in which the evidence is to be used;
3. how the implementation process is *facilitated.*

These three elements are all important in determining the success of the research use. Each element is positioned on a low-to-high continuum. The PARIHS model predicts, in sum, that the most successful implementation will occur when all elements are on the high end of the continuum.

The core tenets of PARIHS can be summarised as follows [14]:

1. 'Evidence' consists of both formal and informal sources of knowledge, including research evidence, clinical experience (including professional craft knowledge), patient preferences and experiences, and local information.
2. Combining and implementing such evidence in practice involves negotiation and development of a shared understanding about the benefits, disbenefits, risks and advantages of the new over the old. This is a dialectical process that requires team effort and careful facilitation. It cannot be achieved by individuals working in isolation.
3. Some contexts are more conducive to the successful implementation of evidence than others. A conducive context includes transformational leaders, features of learning organisations and appropriate monitoring, evaluation and feedback.
4. Facilitators can work with both individuals and teams to enhance the process of implementation. The approach to facilitation, and the role and skill requirements of the facilitator, will be influenced by the *state of preparedness* of an individual or team. This will include their acceptance and understanding of the evidence and the organisational context (resources, culture and values, leadership style and evaluation activity).

The ideal situation for implementing evidence in a team – strong evidence on which all parties agree plus a context that is highly receptive to applying this evidence (i.e. well-resourced and with a culture of improvement) – is rarely found. But, suggests PARIHS, good facilitation can (sometimes but not always) help teams work to obtain stronger evidence, increase the level of consensus around the evidence and work together to strengthen the organisational context.

Figure A.7 shows the PARIHS diagnostic and evaluative grid. Its authors propose that the first step when attempting to implement evidence in a team is to assess both the evidence and the context (including the position, attitude to evidence and learning needs of individual staff members) in a way that allows you to map the team's starting point somewhere on the two-by-two matrix.

If the main issue identified is that staff members are unaware of the evidence (or unaware of how to evaluate it), for example, the main role of the facilitator might be to work with individuals to support relevant learning and personal development. On the other hand, the initial diagnostic assessment might suggest a more task-focused intervention (e.g. assistance with project management or negotiating resources). A facilitator may thus play a range of

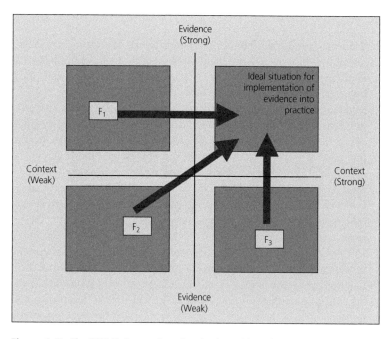

Figure A.7　The PARIHS diagnostic and evaluative grid. F = facilitation. *Source:* Kitson et al. [14]. © Kitson et al.; licensee BioMed Central Ltd. 2008. Open Access article distributed under the terms of the Creative Commons Attribution License (http://creativecommons.org/licenses/by/2.0).

different roles, all concerned with assessment of the situation, assessment of individual, team and workplace readiness, development of change and evaluation strategies, support of the implementation process, coaching and mentoring of the team through the change and monitoring of progress.

The PARIHS team has produced assessment tools that can be used in both the diagnostic and monitoring phases of this process [14], and, more recently, a book-length guide to the assessment and facilitation process [15].

A team in the United States led by Christian Helfrich reviewed the literature on the application of the PARIHS framework [16]. At the time of the review, in 2009, 18 empirical studies had been published. None had used PARIHS in the way the original authors had recommended – to undertake a 'diagnosis' of the evidence–context relationship and plan facilitation accordingly. All had used the framework to aid retrospective analysis. The framework had proved intuitively appealing, easy to understand, flexible and relatively easy to apply to the (mostly qualitative) datasets. But few studies had successfully measured the different dimensions of evidence and context in a quantified and/or reproducible way. Helfrich et al. proposed further refinement of the concepts in the PARIHS framework and its use in prospective studies.

Notwithstanding the many criticisms of PARIHS in the literature, I personally like it a lot. It has what I would call 'face validity' – that is, it seems intuitively sensible that evidence, context and facilitation are all key to implementation, and that they interact. Furthermore, at a broad-brush level, the PARIHS framework is sufficiently flexible to allow its application to many different situations and examples. The lack of published worked examples suggests that PARIHS is not as easy to formalise as was once (perhaps) assumed. My own view is that this is less a limitation of PARIHS than it is a reflection of the fluid and complex nature of team and organisational knowledge. As with the other frameworks introduced in this appendix, it is not a panacea.

Plan–do–study–act (PDSA) cycles

Many people know what the letters in the acronym PDSA mean – but far fewer understand what the words 'plan', 'do', 'study' and 'act' mean in practice or where PDSA fits into a wider change effort. The key point is that a PDSA cycle (or spiral – see Figure A.8) is a tool for undertaking rapid, small-scale tests of change. It is not, in and of itself, a framework for achieving a programme of major structural or cultural change – although such a programme might well include PDSA cycles somewhere. Indeed, having seen PDSA misused by a few senior managers, clinical directors and doctoral students (all with the best of intentions), I would like to propose that PDSA cycles henceforth be referred to as 'rapid and small-scale change assessment loops' (RASCALs).

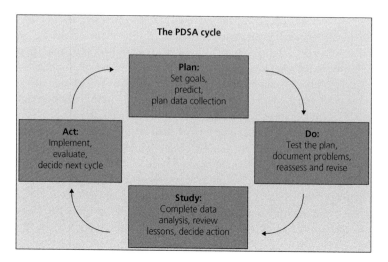

Figure A.8 Plan–do–study–act (PDSA) cycle. *Source:* Langley, G., Nolan, K., Nolan, T., Norman, C., & Provost, L. (1996). *The Improvement Guide: A Practical Approach to Enhancing Organizational Performance.* San Francisco, CA, Jossey-Bass Publishers, pp. 6–11. Reproduced with permission of John Wiley & Sons.

The point about PDSA cycles is that they are experimental and iterative (set out to try something, systematically assess its impact, adjust the approach, try it again – and so on). What you measure and how will depend on the situation, of course (see 'Measurement for Improvement'). The following paragraph sums up the rationale for PDSA cycles and describes how they can also be used as engagement tools to draw staff into the change process so that they quickly feel a part of the effort:

> *Conducting small-scale tests through a 'Plan, Do, Study, Act' (PDSA) cycle provides a useful and safe opportunity to try the idea, reflect on the outcome and then either change the plan or try it on a larger cohort of patients. Each cycle of testing provides new information and evidence about the change idea, which should be captured and shared with others. Through the use of these test cycles, information is provided in a number of different ways, including through observation data that is collected to form evidence about the test and then a thought process which assimilates all that has gone before and identifies a way forward. It can also act as a method to involve others who will be affected by the change.* [12]

In sum, by all means include some PDSA cycles in your plan for implementing EBHC – but make sure you also have an overarching strategy and rationale that is couched in a wider theory or framework.

Process mapping

Anyone who has experienced healthcare recently knows that the process of finding the right health professional for one's problem, undergoing tests, receiving care and monitoring treatment is often extremely complex (so much so that hospitals often employ 'care navigators' just to help patients work out how to get from one part of the system to another and join up all the different elements of their care). As Chapter 4 emphasised, contemporary clinical care is usually a team activity – so it is crucial for those seeking to change care processes to be clear about who does what, in what order.

Process mapping is *a multidisciplinary team activity aimed at producing a map or diagram of all the elements (visits, tasks, procedures and so on) in a patient pathway and the key interfaces involved*. At a hypothetical level, it is a simple process of drawing a box for each step and connecting the boxes in time order. In practice, it may take considerable discussion to surface all the steps and agree on what constitutes a 'step'.

Figure A.9 shows a process map using early breast cancer as an example. Convention dictates that three shapes are used in such maps: an oval for start and end; a diamond for a decision; and a rectangle for all other steps. Many of the steps in Figure A.9 would benefit from further unpacking. For example, a patient embarking on chemotherapy will probably have an initial orientation meeting with a specialist nurse followed by several cycles of chemotherapy and various blood tests and imaging tests to monitor progress. At various stages, the specialist team will need to write to the patient's primary care physician – and so on.

The King's Fund has produced an excellent online resource for process mapping [17].

Stakeholder mapping

It is probably self-evident that when planning a project that affects different groups of people, it is a good idea to list which groups are involved and what each one's agenda and potential input (positive and negative) is. The rationale was well described in an article by Bruga and Varvasovsky a few years ago:

> *Stakeholder analysis can be used to generate knowledge about the relevant actors so as to understand their behaviour, intentions, interrelations, agendas, interests, and the influence or resources they have brought – or could bring – to bear on the decision-making processes. This information can then be used to develop strategies for managing these stakeholders, to facilitate the implementation of specific decisions or organizational objectives, or to understand the policy context and assess the feasibility of future policy directions.* [18]

Appendix A

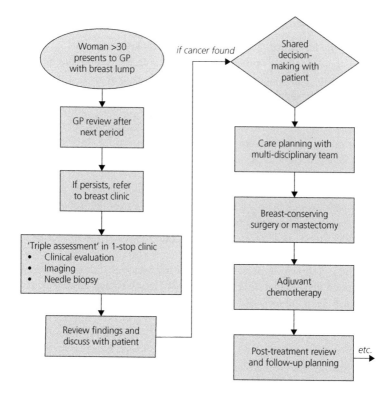

Figure A.9 Simplified process map showing the typical patient journey in early breast cancer.

Some writers depict stakeholder mapping as the construction of a (somewhat crude and subjective) matrix of power and interest. In this approach, stakeholders are divided into those with more or less power (one axis) and more or less interest in the project (the other axis). Those with high power and high interest can be marshalled to support the initiative; those with low power and low interest can be safely ignored; those with high power and low interest can be targeted with information (and perhaps a charm offensive); and so on.

In my experience, stakeholders are not so easily pigeon-holed – and their concerns and qualities have many more dimensions than 'power' and 'interest'. As I explained in Section 2.3, stakeholders come from different cultural worlds and bring different assumptions. These are not necessarily good or bad – just different, and it would be useful to understand where everyone is coming from. Furthermore, supporters can turn into opponents, and vice versa, as a project unfolds.

I personally like to use stakeholder mapping for three tasks. First, an initial stakeholder map (brainstormed on a flip-chart – or even the back of an envelope) can be the starting point for a living database of the contact details of everyone who should be kept informed of the project. This contact list should not be used indiscriminately (different stakeholders will want to keep in touch in different ways; not everyone needs the minutes of the formal meetings and not everyone is going to be following you on Twitter). Second, a stakeholder map should serve to remind you of the complexity and diversity of the system in which your project sits – and the fact that not everyone who has a piece of this project views it in the same way as you do. And third, such a map will be a resource for thinking about how to take forward different aspects of the project (and for seeking to explain why some aspects are not progressing as planned).

In other words, stakeholder maps are useful, but they are not 'tools' in any simple sense. Do not fall into the trap of using stakeholder mapping in a simplistic and overly technical way. Figure A.10 shows a template for organising the information about your stakeholders (but there are many alternative ways of doing it, and none is any more 'correct' than any other).

Value co-creation (adapted for healthcare)

In Section 11.4, in the context of multi-stakeholder health research systems, I briefly referred to Ramaswamy and Ozcan's value co-creation model [19]. This model originally came from the commercial business sector and was intended to prompt companies to think about how to create value for their customers, their staff and their shareholders (and perhaps other groups too). I have adapted it for a healthcare context in Figure A.11. Please do not try to use it in a formulaic way!

Ramaswamy and Ozcan offer four key principles for the co-creation of value across different sectors:

1. Stakeholders will not wholeheartedly participate in the co-creation process unless it *produces value* for them.
2. The best way to co-create value is to *focus on the experiences of all stakeholders*.
3. Stakeholders must be able to *interact directly with one another* (preferably face to face at least some of the time).
4. *Platforms are needed* that allow stakeholders to interact and share their experiences.

As the last of these points indicates, platforms (of various kinds, formal and informal) are a central element of the model, as these are what brings

Appendix A

	Stakeholder group (Add additional columns as appropriate – e.g. Board-level leaders, clinicians, middle managers, patients/carers/families)
Who are the key stakeholders in this group?	
Are they directly involved in the project – if so, how?	
Are they indirectly involved in the project – if so, how?	
Do they have the potential to influence the project – if so, in what way?	
Might they facilitate or create barriers to the project? Why and how might this occur?	
Where/when/how can we link with this stakeholder group?	
What influences this stakeholder group (e.g. are they short of time; do they need money, training etc)?	
Who influences this stakeholder group?	

Figure A.10   Template for a stakeholder map.

stakeholders together. The co-creation process is supported through two key activities, as shown on the right and left sides of Figure A.11, respectively:

1. *Engagement of individuals* (in which people who will be key to the enterprise are engaged and offered support and open-source resources);
2. *Support for enterprise* (which brings organisations together to work on particular projects and programmes and provides a range of resources for this purpose).

In the value co-creation model, capacity-building occurs both through individual training and development *and* through the enterprise process itself.

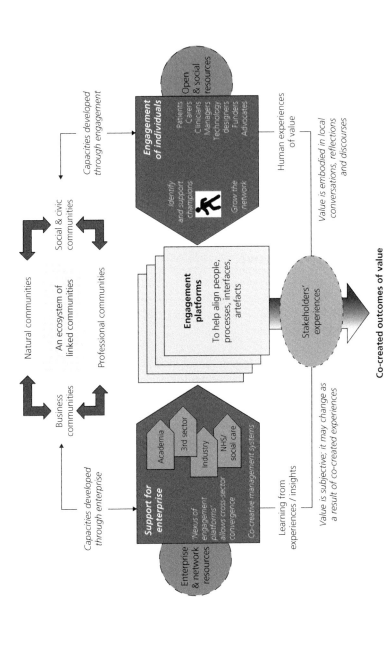

Figure A.11 Value co-creation model. *Source*: Adapted from Ramaswamy & Ozcan [19].

Individuals circulate within and between their various communities of practice (see Section 10.2) – business, professional, natural (e.g. geographical) and civic – sharing experiences and perspectives. Different individuals and different groups value different things. Communication and dialogue – including but not limited to the formal governance processes of the programme(s) – ensure that each stakeholder gets something of what he or she values *and* understands and contributes to what others value.

Although the value co-creation model originated in business studies, it has been applied tentatively to the triple helix of university–industry–government relations, which I described in Section 11.4 [20], and also, in a single instance, to co-creation in a healthcare setting (in Australia) [21]. My own team is currently undertaking additional empirical studies of this model as applied to multi-stakeholder health research systems in the United Kingdom. In a later edition of this book, I hope to report back on whether it proved fit for purpose.

Why, whose, what, how?

Vicky Ward undertook the mammoth task of reviewing 47 published models and frameworks for knowledge mobilisation (i.e. for taking some kind of knowledge and putting it to work somewhere) [22]. She synthesised these into a framework based on four questions:

1. *Why* mobilise knowledge? (e.g. to solve a local problem; to develop new policies or programmes; to implement existing policies or programmes; to change practice; to contribute to the research base);
2. *Whose* knowledge are we talking about (and who might be considered the 'audience' for the knowledge)? (e.g. researchers, practitioners, service users, policymakers or commissioners, service managers);
3. *What* knowledge are we talking about? (e.g. scientific, research-based knowledge; technical know-how; practical wisdom that comes from long years of professional practice; the experiences of staff and patients);
4. *How* might that knowledge be mobilised? (e.g. disseminating formal knowledge; building connections and networks; co-creation).

Vicky's framework is certainly a useful way to begin to get your head round a knowledge mobilisation challenge in your organisation. My own view is that once you have answered all or most of the questions listed here in relation to a particular knowledge mobilisation challenge, you may find you are ready to select a more specific theoretical lens through which to consider a salient angle or framing.

References

1. Howe, C., Randall, K., Chalkley, S., & Bell, D. (2013). Supporting improvement in a quality collaborative. *British Journal of Healthcare Management, 19*, 434–442.
2. Resar, R., Griffin, F.A., Haraden, C., & Nolan, T.W. (2012). Using Care Bundles to Improve Health Care Quality. IHI Innovation Series white paper. Available from: http://www.ihi.org/resources/pages/ihiwhitepapers/usingcarebundles.aspx   (last accessed 14 January 2017).
3. Lennox, L., Green, S., Howe, C., Musgrave, H., Bell, D., & Elkin, S. (2014). Identifying the challenges and facilitators of implementing a COPD care bundle. *BMJ Open Respiratory Research, 1*(1):e000035.
4. King's Fund (2016). Driver Diagrams. Available from: http://www.kingsfund.org.uk/projects/pfcc/driver-diagrams (last accessed 14 January 2017).
5. Institute for Health Improvement (2010). IHI 90-Day Research and Development Process. Available from: http://www.ihi.org/about/Documents/IHI90DayResearchandDevelopmentProcessAug10.pdf (last accessed 14 January 2017).
6. Bate, P., & Robert, G. (2007). *Bringing User Experience to Healthcare Improvement: The Concepts, Methods and Practices of Experience-Based Design*. Abingdon, Radcliffe Publishing.
7. King's Fund (2013). Experience-Based Co-Design Toolkit. Available from: http://www.kingsfund.org.uk/projects/ebcd (last accessed 14 January 2017).
8. Iedema, R., Merrick, E., Piper, D., Britton, K., Gray, J., Verma, R., & Manning, N. (2010). Codesigning as a discursive practice in emergency health services: the architecture of deliberation. *The Journal of Applied Behavioral Science, 46*(1), 73–91.
9. Graham, I.D., Logan, J., Harrison, M.B., Straus, S.E., Tetroe, J., Caswell, W., & Robinson, N. (2006). Lost in knowledge translation: time for a map? *Journal of Continuing Education in the Health Professions, 26*(1), 13–24.
10. NHS Scotland (2016). Measurement for Improvement. Available from: http://www.qihub.scot.nhs.uk/knowledge-centre/quality-improvement-topics/measurement-for-improvement.aspx (last accessed 14 January 2017).
11. Kaplan, R.S., & Norton, D.P. (1996). *The Balanced Scorecard: Translating Strategy into Action*. Cambridge, MA, Harvard Business Press.
12. NHS Institute for Innovation and Improvement. Sustainability Model and Guide. Available from: http://www.qihub.scot.nhs.uk/media/162236/sustainability_model.pdf (last accessed 14 January 2017).
13. Popay, J., & Collins, M. (2014). Public Involvement Impact Assessment Framework. Available from: http://piiaf.org.uk/index.php (last accessed 4 March 2017).
14. Kitson, A.L., Rycroft-Malone, J., Harvey, G., McCormack, B., Seers, K., & Titchen, A. (2008). Evaluating the successful implementation of evidence into practice using the PARiHS framework: theoretical and practical challenges. *Implementation Science, 3*(1), 1.
15. Harvey, G., & Kitson, A. (2015). *Implementing Evidence-Based Practice in Healthcare: A Facilitation Guide*. London, Routledge.
16. Helfrich, C.D., Damschroder, L.J., Hagedorn, H.J., Daggett, G.S., Sahay, A., Ritchie, M., et al. (2010). A critical synthesis of literature on the promoting action on research implementation in health services (PARIHS) framework. *Implementation Science, 5*(1), 82.

17. King's Fund. Process Mapping. Available from: http://www.kingsfund.org.uk/ projects/pfcc/process-mapping (last accessed 14 January 2017).

18. Brugha, R., & Varvasovszky, Z. (2000). Stakeholder analysis: a review. *Health Policy and Planning*, **15**(3), 239–246.

19. Ramaswamy, V., & Ozcan, K. (2014). *The Co-Creation Paradigm*. Stanford, CT, Stanford University Press.

20. Hughes, T. (2014). Co-creation: moving towards a framework for creating innovation in the triple helix. *Prometheus*, **32**(4), 337–350.

21. Greenhalgh, T., Jackson, C., Shaw, S., & Janaiman, T. (2016). Achieving research impact through co-creation in community-based health services: literature review and case study. *The Milbank Quarterly*, **94**(2), 392–429.

22. Ward, V. (2016). Why, whose, what and how? A framework for knowledge mobilisers. *Evidence and Policy*, doi: https://doi.org/10.1332/174426416X14634763278725.

Appendix B Psychological domains and constructs relevant to the implementation of EBHC

Domains	Constructs
1. Knowledge	Knowledge
	Knowledge about condition/scientific rationale
	Schemas + mindsets + illness representations
	Procedural knowledge
2. Skills	Skills
	Competence/ability/skill assessment
	Practice/skills development
	Interpersonal skills
	Coping strategies
3. Social/ professional role and identity	Identity
	Professional identity/boundaries/role
	Group/social identity
	Social/group norms (→ alienation/organisational commitment)
4. Beliefs about capabilities	Self-efficacy: control – of behaviour and material/social environment
	Perceived competence
	Self-confidence/professional confidence
	Empowerment
	Self-esteem
	Perceived behavioural control
	Optimism/pessimism
5. Beliefs about consequences	Outcome expectancies (anticipated regret, appraisal/ evaluation/review)
	Consequents
	Attitudes
	Contingencies
	Reinforcement/punishment/consequences
	Incentives/rewards
	Beliefs
	Unrealistic optimism
	Salient events/sensitisation/critical incidents
	Characteristics of outcome expectancies – physical, social, emotional
	Sanctions/rewards, proximal/distal, valued/not valued, probable/improbable, salient/not salient, perceived risk/threat

(Continued)

How to Implement Evidence-Based Healthcare, First Edition. Trisha Greenhalgh.
© 2018 John Wiley & Sons Ltd. Published 2018 by John Wiley & Sons Ltd.

Domains	Constructs
6. Motivation and goals	Intention; stability of intention/certainty of intention Goals (autonomous, controlled) Goal target/setting Goal priority Intrinsic motivation Commitment Distal and proximal goals Transtheoretical model and stages of change
7. Memory, attention and decision processes	Memory Attention Attention control Decision-making
8. Environmental context and resources	Resources/material resources (availability and management) Environmental stressors Person–environment interaction Knowledge of task environment
9. Social influences (norms)	Social support Social/group norms Organisational development Leadership Team working Group conformity Organisational climate/culture Social pressure Power/hierarchy Professional boundaries/roles Management commitment Supervision Intergroup conflict Champions Social comparisons Identity; group/social identity Organisational commitment/alienation Feedback Conflict – competing demands, conflicting roles Change management Crew resource management Negotiation Social support: personal/professional/organisational, intra/interpersonal, society/community Social/group norms: subjective, descriptive, injunctive norms Learning and modelling
10. Emotion (emotion)	Affect Stress Anticipated regret Fear Burn-out Cognitive overload/tiredness Threat Positive/negative affect Anxiety/depression

Domains	Constructs
11. Behavioural regulation	Goal/target setting
	Implementation intention
	Action planning
	Self-monitoring
	Goal priority
	Generating alternatives
	Feedback
	Moderators of intention–behaviour gap
	Project management
	Barriers and facilitators
12. Nature of the behaviours	Routine/automatic/habit
	Breaking habit
	Direct experience/past behaviour
	Representation of tasks
	Stages of change model

Source: Michie 2005 [1]. Reproduced with permission of BMJ Publishing Group Ltd.

Reference

1. Michie, S., Johnston, M., Abraham, C., Lawton, R., Parker, D., & Walker, A. (2005). Making psychological theory useful for implementing evidence based practice: a consensus approach. *Quality and Safety in Health Care*, **14**(1), 26–33.

Index

Page numbers in *italics* refer to illustrations; those in **bold** refer to tables

How to Implement Evidence-Based Healthcare, First Edition. Trisha Greenhalgh.
© 2018 John Wiley & Sons Ltd. Published 2018 by John Wiley & Sons Ltd.

Printed and bound by CPI Group (UK) Ltd, Croydon, CR0 4YY

14/03/2023

03201475-0001